I0413840

Balance Disorders
A Brief Overview

MR TARIQ KHAN

authorHOUSE®

AuthorHouse™ UK
1663 Liberty Drive
Bloomington, IN 47403 USA
www.authorhouse.co.uk
Phone: 0800.197.4150

Published by AuthorHouse

ISBN: 978-1-5462-9807-6 (sc)
ISBN: 978-1-7283-8380-4 (hc)
ISBN: 978-1-5462-9806-9 (e)

Contents

Preface

I started to develop an interest in balance disorders in 2005. These are complex disorders, and I was met with constant challenges in dealing with these patients. This flared up my interest in this field. My audiology and physiotherapy colleagues were very helpful and showed a lot of enthusiasm, and we started a dedicated balance clinic. The benefits to these patients with these clinics were very encouraging. I also started an awareness campaign in the primary care, and with the help of a very helpful young patient of mine, I started to mentor a patient awareness group.

I also took a keen interest in teaching. This prompted me to write guidelines for the junior doctors in the department and also modify and write patient information leaflets, which are very popular with staff and patients. In fact, it was these guidelines which kept extending, and I then thought of compiling them in a book.

There are many excellent books and a lot of literature is available on these topics. This small book is an effort to simplify this complex topic. Its aim is to provide basic knowledge and understanding of this subject at the level of a junior registrar, primary care physicians and trainee audiologists. This can be used as a simplified guideline to deal with patients. Diagnosis of balance problems can be quite challenging. It is very common practice with number of practitioners at junior level to send patients for unnecessary balance lab investigations without understanding the rationale and limitations of these tests. I believe this book can be used as a quick reference to solve these dilemmas.

Tariq Khan FRCS(ORL) VM-AIB
Certification balance management (American Institute of Balance)
ENT specialist with special interest in balance disorders
Hull and East York Teaching Hospital Trust
Hull,UK

Introduction

Balance disorders are very common. About 20 per cent of eighteen-to sixty-four-year-olds report dizziness in the preceding year, and of those reporting resulting handicap from their dizziness, only one in four have received treatment. It is also the commonest symptom presenting to GPs in those over seventy-five. It is often chronic, poorly diagnosed, and undertreated.

Tariq Khan has put together an easy-to-read introduction covering the important aspects of physiology and investigation, followed by a summary of the common conditions a physician might encounter. Identifying the diagnosis—and not just the symptom of dizziness—is key to good patient care.

This work will provide a very useful guide for those wishing to gain an introduction to the fascinating world of dizziness and balance.

Professor Peter Rea
Consultant ENT Surgeon
University Hospitals of Leicester
Director, Leicester Balance Centre
Honorary Professor of Balance Medicine
De Montfort University, Leicester, UK

Anatomy and Physiology of Vestibular System

There are three fundamental components of human vestibular system.

1. Sensory input.
   - Visual
   - From joints and musculoskeletal system
   - Peripheral vestibular system

2. Integration/processing of senses in CNS to create appropriate response.
   This is achieved by three main pathways:
   - Coordination between inner ear and eyes. VOR (vestibular ocular reflex). It generates eye movements that keep vision clear with head movements.
   - Coordination between the inner ear and spine. VSR (vestibular spinal reflex). It generates body movements to stabilise the posture.
   - Another type of reflex has also been described, called VCR (vestibular collic reflex). It acts on neck musculature to stabilise the head.

3. Performing motor commands.
   The sensory input from visual, proprioceptive, and vestibular receptors are processed in the cerebellum and finely

adjusted by higher cortical centres. These adjustments are very adaptive and have great plasticity.

There is innate capability to adapt in the higher centres and repair. In fact, in patientswho have unilateral vestibular failure, and who are otherwise fit and well, it can be very hard to detect the damage after a year. This forms the basis of rehabilitation in vestibular disorders.

Peripheral vestibular system is housed in the otic capsule that lies in the temporal bone on each side. It consists of membranous labyrinth and the bony labyrinth.

Semicircular Canals

There are three semi circular canals called posterior, lateral (horizontal), and superior (anterior). These canals are arranged at almost right angles to each other and in the same plane to the opposite ear. They sense the angular motion and are most sensitive in the direction of rotation in their own plane. Rotation in one plane will be excitatory to the canal on one side and inhibitory to the other side. In certain angles, the canals on both sides work together to facilitate the sensations.

The horizontal canal senses the rotation in horizontal plane. Oblique head movements are sensed by the anterior canal on one side and the posterior canal on the other side. Head down movement will stimulate both anterior canals on one side and inhibit both posterior canals on the opposite side. Head up movement does the opposite.

Each canal has a dilated end called the ampulla that contains hair cells and a divider called the cupula. As a result of the head movements, the endolymph exerts pressure on the cupula, resulting in its deflection. This leads to bending of hair cells, thus generating the action potential down to vestibular nerve.

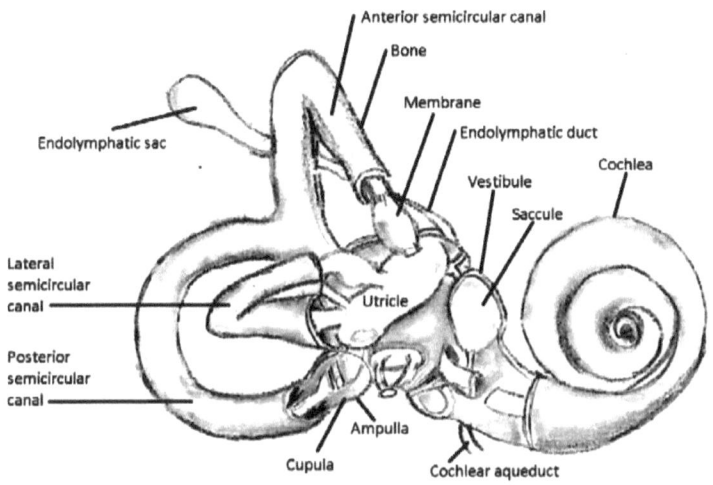

Figure 1. Membranous labyrinth.

It is important to understand that the semicircular canal afferents constantly discharge, even in the absence of any rotation. The cupular deflection increases the rate of discharge in the direction of angle of the canal and decreases the neural activity in opposite direction. On both sides, the level of neural activity is in equilibrium at all times (i.e., at rest or during an activity). The brain senses the direction of rotation by detecting change in this ratio.

In vestibular failure or hypofunction, the neural discharge decreases on that side, and the brain assumes that head is rotating. This explains why patients with vestibular hypofunction experience sense of rotation or vertigo even when the head is stationary.

Otolithic Organs

There are two otolithic organs on each side. They sense the linear acceleration of the head. The utricle is oriented in the horizontal plane, making it sensitive to horizontal acceleration, and the saccule is placed almost vertical so it is stimulated by vertical motions.

The hair cells of otolithic organs are loaded with calcium crystals called otoconia. With acceleration in either plane, the gelatinous membranecontaining these crystals is 'left behind'. This results in generation of action potential in the vestibular nerve.

This specific organization of canals and otolithic organs keeps the check on balance control in both dynamic and static body movements and postures.

Most of the vestibular tests are directed towards testing the horizontal canals. So effectively, we mostly test one-fifth of balance organs. This explains why the vestibular tests are negative in many patients with significant clinical issues.

Gaze Control System

Vestibular nuclei are located in the brainstem, where they relay in the medial longitudinal fasciculus. Here they reach the nuclei of the third, fourth, and sixth nerves. These connections form the basis of conjugate eye movements in relation to head movements called vestibulo ocular reflex (VOR).

The function of gaze control system to is to keep the object of interest in the focus. VOR is active when the head is in motion and other systems (smooth pursuit, saccades, and optokinetic) are active when the object is moving. Therefore it is important in normal, day-to-day life for these systems to coordinate, especially when both the head and the object of interest are moving (e.g., keeping everything in focus while walking in crowded areas).

VOR

VOR stabilises the gaze during the head movements. All objects around us are always kept in sharp focus irrespective of whether the head is static or moving. This is due to VOR. It works by moving the eyes with the same speed as the head movements but in opposite direction.

The clearest image of any object is formed in the centre of fovea. During any motion, the image slips to periphery, causing it to blur. Movement of two degrees from centre will lead to 50 per cent decrease in visual acuity.

To keep the image in centre of the fovea, the eyes make corrective motions called nystagmus, which have a slow and a quick phase. VOR keeps the image central with a slow phase of eye (opposite to head movements).

In patients with vestibular disorders, VOR is affected in most cases. This leads to destabilization of the gaze-fixing mechanism, and patients find their mobility is compromised, especially in high-velocity head movements (e.g.,walking andrunning). It can also affect the visual acuity. In patients with vestibular failure, the visual acuity can drop up to four lines.

VOR actively stabilises the vision, however there are certain situations where the normal VOR needs to be suppressed. This is needed when one wants to focus on object that is rotating at high speed (e.g., following a ball by moving the head and eyes in order to keep the ball focused, like watching a tennis match).

VOR suppression involves visual cues and voluntary target fixation. This is a function of central nervous pathways. In central lesions, VOR suppression is affected.

Practically, this means that lesion of one system does affect the other. That is, lesions of central system will affect peripheral system.

Other Systems of Gaze Control

Smooth Pursuit
This system allows eyes to track slowly moving objects in the visual field. It uses foveal stimulation. It declines with object speed, age, sedative medicines, and lesions of the cerebellum.

Saccades
In this system, high-velocity object are tracked, which may be in or out of visual field. They are the refixating eye movements. Some of them are involuntary (e.g., eye movements in response to a sound).

Optokinetic
This system is like smooth pursuit but uses full field stimulation. It uses peripheral retinal stimulation.

The function of all these systems, together with VOR, is to keep object of interest in focus. VOR is active when the head is moving, whereas other systems (smooth persuit, saccades, optokinetic) are active when the object is moving.

The cerebellum plays a central role in higher controls of balance. It modulates the final motor activity and triggers vestbulospinal reflex (VSR) and vestibulo colic reflex (VCR),which stabilise the posture and the head, respectively.

There is such a close relation between vestibular and ocular mobility that examination of the ocular system makes the basis of assessment of vestibular system.

Here's a table to summarise the eye movements.

Table 1.1

Eye Movements/ Pathway	Function	Abnormality	Possible Lesion
VOR	Stabilise gaze during head movements	Horizontal nystagmus	Peripheral vestibular
Smooth Pursuit	Tracking of slow-moving object (foveal stimulation)	Saccadic persuit	Central (cerebellum, brainstem)
Saccades	Tracking fast-moving object/ refixation on new object	Late saccades or disconjugate movements	Central
Optokinetic	Sense movements with peripheral vision	Absent or asymmetric	Central

Posture Control System

Posture control has two functions in the body.

1. Maintaining posture against gravity.
2. Orientation of the body.

It is the function of the brain to maintain an upright posture in static or mobile situations by integrating the sensations from vestibular organs, visual cues, and the somatosensory system. Specific muscle groups(e.g., spinal, hip, leg, and ankle) are responsible for carrying out these functions. The main object is to keep the body balanced on its base of support.

In human beings, the development of balance system is quite complex. A child takes almost twelve to eighteen months to learn to walk. Our base of support is a small area where feet come in contact with the surface. In daily life activities, balance is maintained by constantly adjusting centre of gravity (COG) in relation to base of support. Larger COG displacements will need a quick step or a stumble to prevent falling.

We employ three different strategies in relation to our base of support to keep centre of gravity (COG) in line. This keeps the body balanced and prevents a fall.

1. Ankle Strategy:When the base is firm with a rigid body, the 'ankle strategy'is used to adjust minor changes in posture.
2. Hip Strategy: In cases where base is not predictable, larger adjustments are needed, and then the 'hip strategy'is employed.
3. Step Strategy: In very large shift of base or body, the 'step strategy'is involved. We step forward or backwards to prevent falling.

This is an important concept because correct assessment of these functions in a patient will help to plan appropriate vestibular rehabilitation.

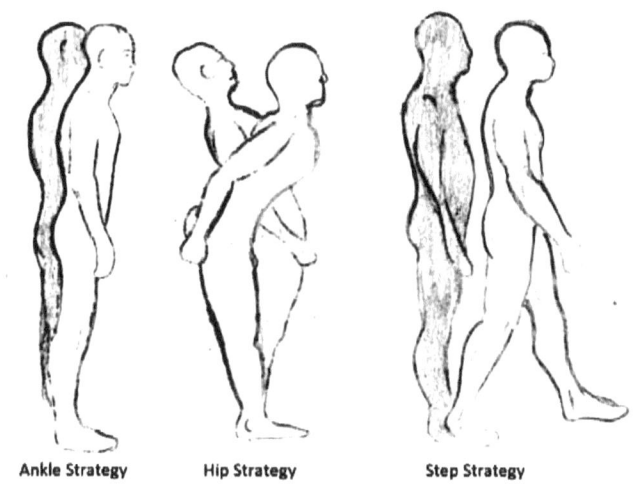

Ankle Strategy   Hip Strategy   Step Strategy

Figure 2. Schemetic diagram of strategies for posture control.

Sensory Conflict

It is the sensory conflict in the orientation of the balance system that causes a sense of imbalance or vertigo. In unilateral vestibular failure, there will be abnormal or reduced discharge from the neurons. This gives the perception that the body is moving. However, the brain immediately realises with spatial orientation that this is not the case, andit tries to correct it, followed by another such cycle. This induces imbalance or vertigo depending on the severity and extent of lesion. It can happen in static or in ambulatory situations.

It is difficult to explain why it is accompanied by nausea or vomiting. One of the theories is that with a certain degree of sensory conflict, the brain thinks that the body has been poisoned, and so it triggers the vomiting centre to get rid of the stomach's contents.

So in short, the vestibular system through semicircular canals (by sensing angular motion), and the otolithic organs (linear- and gravity-related motions) produce postural control and oculomotor responses. These responses are kept in check by the cerebellum and cortical areas to fully integrate the body's response to a given task according to a particular situation, time, and place.

All these systems seamlessly work at the subconscious level. In situations where a deficiency is encountered at any level, either peripheral (vestibular organs, procrioctive, visual) or central (cerebellum or cortical), compensatory processes kick in. For example, with vestibular issues patients start to use more visual cues. In vestibular hypofunction, it becomes very difficult for patients to walk in dark areas or more reliance on sensory input from joints including feet (difficulty in balance and posture control on uneven floor or stairs). This can be detected in an examination room in tests like the Romberg or Untenberger stepping tests. There is huge plasticity in all these systems, and this can be successfully manipulated by appropriate rehabilitation techniques in the treatment of balance disorders.

Assessment of Patients with Balance Disorders

ℰ❧

The presentation of balance disorders can be complex and multifactorial. A careful history plays a pivotal role. It is not unusual for patients to present in the balance clinic after prolonged sufferings and multiple consultations with a variety of specialities. Detailed history with the stress on chronology of the symptoms is essential. In some situations, it can become difficult for a clinician to extract all the facts within the limited time available in the clinics. Therefore it will be a fruitful practice to ask patients to fill up a balance questionnaire before they come in the clinic room. Every physician can follow their own method in this. It is our practice to send the balance questionnaire to patients with the appointment. They fill it up in their own time without any stress. This helps the patients because they would fully outline their symptoms, and it also helps physicians to build a comprehensive picture.

A standardised questionnaire is available called Dizziness Handicap Inventory (DHI). It is very useful because it outlines the salient features in the history, and it can be used to assess the functional disabilities of the patients. It incorporates a scoring system through which a patient's progress during the course of treatment can be effectively assessed.

The scoring system helps to build up the confidence of the patient. It is not uncommon to find that patients feel at times their treatment is getting stagnant. This is due to the fact that when their symptoms start improving, the expectations become higher, and the patient thinks that progress is not as swift as it should be. In these situations, one can objectively prove to patients that their scoring is improving by constantly assessing them on the DHI scoring system. This boosts their own confidence and trust in the therapist. These factors play an important role during the course of treatment.

An attempt to differentiate between the peripheral and central causes of dizziness will always be a key factor in assessment.

History

History has a pivotal role in diagnosis. Some important features are outlined below to build a more organised approach.

Presentation can be varied, to say the least. It depends a lot on the patient's ability to describe his or her symptoms. In many instances, it can become a challenge for the physician to extract accurate history. On the other hand, it can be frustrating for the patient to give a precise account of their symptoms.

In the beginning, let the patient tell the story. In an interesting study, it was shown that most patients will tell whatever they want within the first ninety seconds of consultation.

A patient may use different terms: light-headed, spinning, feeling off balance, walking on cotton wool, feeling drunk.

It is important in the course of the history to determine the accurate chronology of the events. For example, start the history from the first ever episode of dizziness. This gives an insight into causation and longevity of the issue, which may be otherwise missed. Many patients at the first consultation talk about the recent episodes which may be a flare-up of the balance issue, and they might have overlooked the same problem which has happened earlier. It is important for the physician to be aware of this fact to take the grips of the events from very beginning.

It is also imperative to ask whether there has been:

1. Single episode of acute vertigo (vestibular neuronitis, infective, vascular lesion)
2. Recurrent episodic vertigo (migraine, Ménière's)
3. Positional (BPPV, migraine)
4. Constant imbalance, light-headed, or vertigo. Neurological disorders like Parkinson's, myolopathy, neuropathies, cerebellar disease, chronic drug toxicity. Psychological.

Duration

The duration of the presentation can commonly be assessed as under:

- Seconds: BPPV, arrhythmias
- Minutes – Hours: Ménière's, migraine
- Days: Vest neuronitis (usually initial attack), stroke
- Permanent: Vest failure (B/L, U/L), psychogenic, MS

It is important, and sometimes it can be tricky to get accurate information from the patients. They can get confused between symptoms resulting from actual vertigo episodes and after-effects they experience. A patient may say he was dizzy for days, but careful interview will reveal that the actual episode was for a few hours, and they did not feel well for few days. This can be vital fact in the history.

Associated Symptoms

The history of associated symptoms is the keystone to establish the diagnosis. It will help to narrow the suspected diagnosis and will determine the direction of further investigations.

- Photophobia, visual aura, headaches, travel sickness: migraine
- Hearing loss, tinnitus, ear fullness: Ménière's
- Syncope, blackouts: Vaso vagal, arrhythmias, orthostatic hypotension
- Loss of consciousness: Epilepsy, hypoglycaemia (rarely associated with vestibular issues)
- Palpitations, panic, trembling: Anxiety
- Diplopia, dysarthria, paresis, memory loss or other neurological deficit:

Space occupying lesions or other acute or chronic neurological deficits, posterior fossa pathology

Past Medical History

The importance of this cannot be overshadowed. Particular stress is to be given on cardiovascular problems, mental health status (diagnosed or undiagnosed anxiety-related problems), and musculoskeletal problems. All these factors play a huge role in reaching a diagnosis and formulating a management plan.

Drug History

It is interesting to note that one-third of all medications in BNF have a side effect of dizziness.

The list of medicines causing dizziness is exhaustive. The common and important drugs which can cause vertigo are as follows.

Anticonvulsants:	Lamotrigine, carbamazapine (common in children)
Antihypertensive:	Amlodipine
Antidepressants:	Mitrazipine
Antibiotics:	Ciprofluxacine, augmentin
Diuretics:	Frusemide
Statin:	Atrovastatin

Examination

Ideally, the clinical examination should start when the patient walks in the clinic room. It will be a good practice to call the patient in the room yourself to watch her gait and the manner with which she maintains posture. During the interview, assessment of the patient's mental health status will be a brownie point.

Clinical examination can be modified according to the patient's symptoms, age, and any other related issues. For example, an elderly patient with coexisting morbidities presenting with typical history of BPPV may not need a full neuro-otological workup.

A specialist balance clinic does not need extensive resources. This service can be provided with a basic ENT outpatient setup. It will be useful to have a facility for auroscopy, tuning forks (512Hz and 256Hz), a couch, and a piece of foam(2×2 feet) within the examining room. Frenzel glasses or having VNG within a clinic room can be of great help.

A protocol of assessment should be developed in order to carry it out smoothly and without leaving a chance to miss any clinical finding.

Examination

Generally, the examination will start from full oto-neurogical workup. That will include otoscopy, tests for cranial nerves, and cerebellar-limb tests. One useful, simple test for sensory input is to apply a 250Hz tuning fork to sole of a foot, especially the heel area. In diabetics, this may be the first sensory neuropathy.

Eye Examination

The relationship between the visual and the vestibular systems is intricate. There are fixed pathways between extra ocular muscles and the vestibular system. These tests will provide an insight into differentiation between central and peripheral problems, and they can localise the peripheral site of lesion.

An eye examination is mandatory in the balance system assessment.

It is also important to perform the tests in a particular order because some of the tests (e.g.,head shake or head thrust) can make some people very dizzy. This may make it difficult to carry out the rest of the examination.

Nystagmus

Nystagmus and its interpretation can be quite tricky, and in many cases it is not easy to follow. The observations to record in nystagmus are as follows.

1. Latency
2. Duration
3. Fixation
4. Fatigability

The differences between central and peripheral nystagmus are listed in the table.

	Central	Peripheral
Latency	Nil	2–15seconds
Duration	Prolonged (up to 120seconds)	Upto 30seconds
Fatigability	Usually not	Always
Fixation	No suppression when fixation removed (e.g., Frenzel glasses)	Always suppressed when fixation removed
Direction	Vertical, horizontal	Horizontal, rotatory
Vertigo	No associated vertigo	Vertigo present

Tests for Nystagmus

Eye Movements	Method	Results	Interpretation
Spontaneous Nystagmus	Fix on a target in neutral gaze	a. No nystagmus b. Jerk nystagmus • Fixed direction, fatigable, increase when fixation taken away(Frenzel glasses) a. Direction changing, Non-fatigable b. Pendular	• Normal • Peripheral • Central • Congenital
Gaze-evoked Nystagmus	Ask to hold gaze 20–30 degrees for 10seconds	• No nystagmus • Horizontal • Vertical or in all direction	• Normal • Peripheral • Central

Smooth Persuit	Ask to track finger movements from 45 degrees on one side to 45 degrees to the other	• Smooth eye movements • Saccadic • Irregular	• Normal • Central • Age related, medications
Saccades	Ask to alternate gaze between fingers	• Accurate, conjugate • Overshoot, undershoot	• Normal • Central
Head Thrust	Ask to fix gaze and thrust head 20–30 degrees	• No loss of fixation • Refixation saccades	• Normal • Peripheral
Head Shake	Ask to close eyes and then shake head at 2Hz for 30seconds	• No nystagmus • Horizontal • Vertical	• Normal • Peripheral • Central

Tests for Posture

Posture assessment should start as the patient walks into the examination room, or even before, to see the gait and support she may need as she mobilisesherself from the waiting area to the consulting room.

Gait

As the patient walks in the room, assess how he or she is maintaining the gait. There are eight basic pathological gaits attributed to neurological conditions.

1. Hemiplegic gait: Hemiplgiaon affected side circumduction of legs with upper limb flexed and/or no swing of arms.
2. Spastic diaplegic: Cerebral palsy (hemiplegia on both sides), walk on tiptoes with flexed arms.
3. Parkinson gait: Universal flexion of body with small shuffling steps.
4. Ataxic: MS, trauma,alcohol abuse, stroke, tumours;broad base with staggering. May fall on side of lesion.
5. Choreiform: Basal ganglia disorders. Irregular, jerky involuntary movements of upper and lower limbs.
6. Sensory: Cerebellar dysfunction. Stamping foot to get vibration/sensations in the body. Falls in dark or onuneven floor.
7. Myopathic: Also called waddling gait. It is due to weak pelvic muscle, and patient tends to lean the body to the opposite side of his step.
8. Neuropathic: In peripheral neuropathies, especially with foot drop. High stepping to avoid toes coming in contact with ground first.

All of the above gaits have specific presentation and represent lesions in the specific areas of brain. Patients with these gaits can present with balance issues. Recognition of these will be helpful in the diagnosis and the management.

The patient with unilateral vestibular failure initially will present with a wide base gait for a few days. In the case of a bilateral failure, this type of gait will prolong for many weeks or months.

The Romberg Test

This test is performed under six different conditions. Each condition is to be tested for at least twenty seconds.

(1) Ask the patient to stand with feet togetherwith eyes open.

(2) Ask the patient to stand with feet together with eyes closed.

(3) Ask the patient to stand tandem (take a step forward) with eyes open.

(4) Ask the patient to stand tandem with eyes closed.

(5) Ask the patient to stand on the foam with eyes open.

(6) Ask the patient to stand on the foam with eyes closed.

It is useful to divide this test into separate conditionsbecause this helps to more accurately evaluate clinical conditions. A normal person will be able to perform all six conditions successfully. A person with vestibular deficit will find conditions 5,6, and 7 (described below) difficult.

Results

- Minimum or slight sway (under 15 degrees) on eye closure. Normal
- Excessive sway (more than 15 degrees; Positive Romberg). Proprioception issues. (Also, it could be positive in acute unilateral or acute bilateral vestibular failures.)

Rationale: This test is for the posterior column integrity and vestibular deficits. Patients with sensory deficits (e.g., due to arthritis or diabetes) use more visual cues to maintain the posture. When they are asked to close their eyes, they will start swaying. It is not a test for the cerebellar lesions. With cerebellar problems, patients will sway even when the eyes are open.

The Unterberger (Fukuda) Stepping Test—Condition 7

The patient is asked to clasp the hands or spread arm forward and then march on the same spot with eyes closed for twenty to thirty seconds.

Result: Patients will rotate 45 degree or more to the side of the lesion in vestibular failures.

Rationale: In this test, the patient's visual and sensory compensations are taken away, and so they start rotating to the side of the lesion without realising. Patients with acute or bilateral vestibular failure will find it very hard to perform the test. This in fact is quite a reliable test for unilateral compensated or partially compensated vestibular failures.

The Dix Hallpike Test

This is diagnostic positional test for BPPV.

Method: Ask the patient to sit on the couch, positioning him in a way that when he lies down, his head should be making a 30-degree angle to the body in a horizontal plane. Turn the patient's head towards one side and ask him to lie down quickly, flat on the couch. Look for nystagmus (type, latency, duration, direction). Repeat on the other side. Repeating the test will fatigue the response. It is recommended to do the test early in the morning. Some people suggest that in patients with a positive history and a negative hall pike test, you should repeat the test after a head shake for 20seconds at 2Hz.

Result:
- No nystagmus or dizziness: Normal
- Geotropic (fast component towards the ground)rotatory nystagmus: Posterior canal BPPV of same side.

- Ageotropic (fast component away from the ground): Possible lateral canalithiasis. (In this case, there may not be any latent period, and duration will be longer.)
- Vertical or non-fatigable (central; e.g., Arnold Chiari Malformation). Sometimes central lesions produce exaggerated response to Hallpike Test with severe dizziness and vomiting. Such patients should always have an MRI scan.

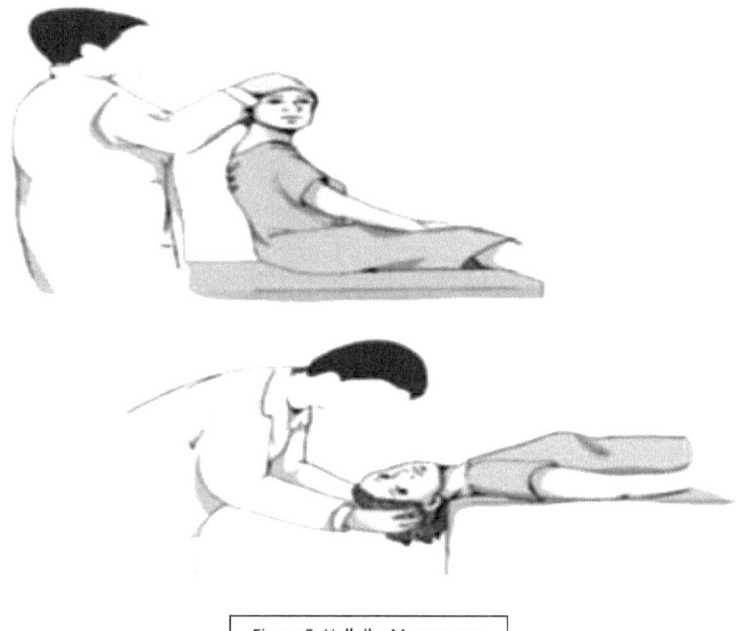

Figure 3. Hallpike Manoeuvre.

Rationale: Each semicircular canal is connected to a specific extra ocular muscle to stabilise the gaze (e.g.,the posterior canal activates the ipsilateral superior oblique and contra lateral inferior rectus, leading to rotatory eye movements). In pathological stimulation of canals, specific nystagmus is induced, which guides towards the diagnosis.

Cerebellar Limb Test

These tests are part of a full neuro-otological workup.

Method: Finger-nose test, heel-shin, rapid alternating motions.

Results:
- Accurate movements   Normal
- Dysmetria, dysdiadochokinesia   Central

Investigations of Patients with Balance Disorders

∾

A detailed and thorough history should lead to the diagnosis in a majority of cases (almost 80–85 per cent). Clinical examination and the investigations will aid in confirming the diagnosis, and in some cases they provide help in establishing the involvement of other systems. There is a very long list of the tests that could be carried out, but the choice of the test will be determined by the presenting complaints or signs elicited on the clinical examination.

Patients with acute symptoms, especially with the first episode, may have a different rationale of approach to the problem. The presentation at times can be difficult to distinguish from posterior fossa pathology, and so a possibility of the cerebrovascular event should be kept in mind.

Presenting with long-term balance issue in routine balance clinic will need evaluation with a different perspective. As mentioned earlier, a patient's general outlook, existing co-morbidities, and age factor need to be taken in consideration when planning for the haematological, radiological tests, or balance lab workup. As a golden rule for every investigation, one has to have a rationale and clear thinking about how that particular test can help in the short- or long-term management of that patient.

The interpretation of balance tests is very complex. Here, an attempt has been made to simplify the basic understanding of these tests.

Pure Tone Audiometry

Most of the patients seen in balance clinic do have some aural symptoms, and so audiometry is necessary in a majority of patients. It is important to find out:

- The type of hearing loss, if any (sensorineural or conductive)
- If sensory neural, then which frequencies (Ménière's is usually low-frequency, fluctuating loss)
- Asymmetry of hearing loss (which will help to outline further investigations, such as MRI, to rule out acoustic neuroma)

Electronystagmography (ENG) and Videonystagmography (VNG)

One of the primary purposes of vestibular apparatus is to control the gaze control. The assessment of movements of the eyes can be used to determine the activities of the peripheral vestibular system and its central connections. ENG will record the corneal-retinal potential by placing electrode near to eyes. These recordings can be carried out with eyes close or open, or in a darkened or lightened room.

The preferred method is videonystagmography (VNG). The difference between ENG and VNG is the method to record the eye movements. ENG is an indirect method of recording. It records the muscle response from eye movements by placing electrode around eyes. VNG, on the other hand, directly records the eye movements with the integrated cameras in the goggles.

It is important to note that assessment of the vestibular system by ENG/VNG recording is significantly limited. The recordings are mainly from the horizontal canal. The information from the vertical canal and otolith organs are very restricted. In fact, only one-fifth of the balance system is put to the test. This explains why patients with significant vertigo symptoms may have normal ENG/VNG results. It is rare that VNG findings will change the pathway of management outlined after clinical diagnosis. This test should not be requested in anticipation that results may change the course of management. It should be read in conjunction with other tests like rotational chair, video head impulse (VHiT), and the posturography. Normal VNG will rule out the central oculomotor involvement but cannot completely rule out peripheral system involvement. However, VNG can prove to be a useful tool in confirmation of the site of lesion.

Indications of ENG/VNG

- To further evaluate and confirm abnormalities in smooth pursuit and saccades seen on clinical examination.
- Long standing and recurrent balance issues.

ENG or Indirect Recording

- Electrodes are placed at the lateral canthus of each eye and one on the forehead (common electrode). One electrodes is placed above the eye and one below the eye.

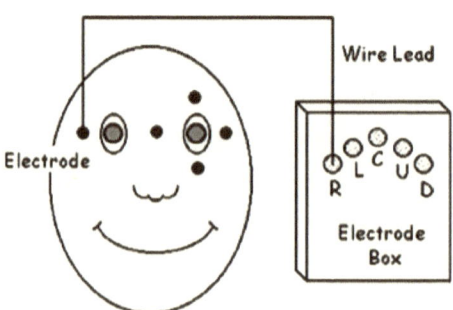

Figure 4. Electrode placement.

VNG or Direct Method

The patient is asked to wear goggles incorporating the cameras to record eye movements. The test is then performed by recording eye movements.

Oculomotor Tests

These tests are performed to assess the abnormalities of central ocular motor controls in the cerebellum and brain stem.

Smooth Pursuit
- This is the most sensitive of all oculomotor tests.
- Abnormality will indicate possible vertibulo-cerebellar region involvement.

Saccades:
- Less sensitive.
- Can provide differentiation between the brain stem and the cerebellum.

Gaze Fixation:
- May provide general suggestions about cerebellar or brain stem involvement.

Optokinetic:
- Least sensitive because it involves both smooth pursuit and saccadic system.

Other VNG Tests
- Spontaneous Nystagmus:
  - The purpose is to record the eye movements when fixation is removed and there are no provocative head movements.
  - Direction-fixed nystagmus indicatesperipheral vestibular pathology.

- Positional Nystagmus:
  - Positional nystagmus is produced by central or peripheral lesions.
  - It should be looked in conjunction with oculomotor study.

- Dix Hallpike:
  - Well-known manoeuvre in clinical examination for BPPV.
  - It is part of routine VNG.

- Caloric Test (Barany's Caloric Test):
  - It is the only test in the battery of VNG workup that can measure labyrinthine function.
  - It can lateralise the peripheral lesion.
  - The air or fluid is typically 7 degrees Celsius above and below the body temperature (i.e., 44 degreesand 30 degrees) and are run in the external auditory canal for 30–40seconds. This change in temperature stimulates the horizontal canal endolymph, producing typical nystagmus.
  - An acronym to remember the direction of nystagmus is COWS (cold opposite, warm same)
  - Maximum slow phase velocity (MSPV) is measured for both sides. Absent or weak response indicates hypofunction of the labyrinth.
  - Direction and strength of nystagmus noted. If direction of nystagmus is stronger on one side, it is called directional preponderance (DP).
  - DP is thought to be due to asymmetric peripheral function without adequate central compensation.

Calculation of Canal Paresis (%) and Directional Preponderance(%):

1. Canal Paresis:

$$\frac{Rw+Rc-Lw+Lc}{Rw+Rc+Lw+Lc} \times 100$$

2. Directional Preponderance:

$$\frac{Rw+Lc-Lw+Rc}{Rw+Rc+Lw+Lc} \times 100$$

- The caloric test is a comparative study of both labyrinths. A difference of more than 20–25 per cent is taken as significant.
- Limitations of the caloric test:
  - It only tests one-fifth of the balance system.
  - During the test, the vestibular system is stimulated by 0.002–0.004Hz. This is a very low frequency movement, which means a single head rotation every five minutes. It is not physiological and is below the level at which normal VOR works.
  - This means results of this test alone cannot completely rule out or rule in any vestibular pathology.
- It should be read in conjunction with other tests and clinical findings.

Rotational Chair Test
- It is the test for horizontal canal VOR. In this test. the vestibular system is stimulated at 1.0–1.2 Hz.
- The two major indication of the rotational chair are:
  1. To test peripheral vestibular system for confirmation of results of VNG tests.
  2. To monitor the patient undergoing chemical labrinthectomy.
- It can also be used in following situations.

- o In cases where caloric testing cannot be done (e.g.,narrow or absent external auditory canal).
  - o When there is disparity in VNG results (e.g., normal results with symptomatic patients).
- In suspected bilateral canal paresis.

Method

- Electrodes are placed, one on each lateral canthus (for horizontal canal) and one on the forehead. These electrodes are connected with the computer.
- The chair is rotated four different ways to provide the stimulus for VOR.
  - o Constant Rotation. Nystagmus is noted in acceleration and deceleration.
  - o Impulse Angular Acceleration. Chair is rotated in one direction and then stopped suddenly. Advantage is that both sides can be tested.
  - o Step Angular Acceleration. Impulse test is repeated but with stepwise change in frequency of rotation. This is done so the patient cannot predict the next move, thus helping to validate the readings.
  - o Sinusoidal Rotation. Rotating patient in alternating direction and with unpredictable change in frequency.

Results:

- Four parameters are taken.
  1. Gain: It is the ratio of amplitude of eye movement to the amplitude of head movement. (No gain in severe cases.)
     - It is $1^0/s^2$ in normal individual and $6-7^0/s^2$ in disease.
     - It gives indication of general responsiveness of the vestibular system.

- It can be influenced by mechanical or neurological restriction in eye movements.
- The principal use of gain measure is to confirm bilateral vestibular failure, which would be initially picked up by caloric test.

2. Phase: Time relationship between head movements and reflexive eye response. (To determine whether any phase lag is present.)

- Normally, eye movements are equal to or lead the head movement. In vestibular failure with no or little compensation, the eyes trail behind; this is called phase lag.
- Phase lag helps in verifying the other tests of VOR.

3. Symmetry: Comparison of slow component of nystagmus of both sides (right and left).

4. Time Constant: It is a measure of time required for VOR gain to decrease. (Typically, exponential decrease by 63 per cent is noted in one second when rotational chair is suddenly stopped.)

- It is reduced in vestibular dysfunction.

Limitations
- It is very expensive equipment and so is not available in all centres.
- As with other tests, the rotational chair test cannot be read alone to reach a confirmatory diagnosis because it mainly tests horizontal canal.

Video Head Impulse Test (VHiT)

- Dr Halmagy and Dr Curthoys described a method of high-frequency test (2–3 Hz) for VOR which simulates the day-to-day head movements. It provides quick and precise information about VOR.

- It is the measurement of VOR in response to head movements.
- Frequency measured in VHiT is closest to physiologic head movements.
- One of the major advantages is that all six canals can be tested.
- It can be done as a reliable bedside test because it is very quick and accurate.
- Patients with vestibular deficit will exhibit catch-up saccade and gain of head in relation to eye movements. VHiT will reliably record this deficit.

Indications

- It is to test VOR. It is easy, quick, and repeatable without much anxieties and discomfort to patients as compared to caloric test.
- It can be used as a reliable bedside test for an immediate result.
- It can be done in ten minutes.

Method

- The hardware includes lightweight goggles with integrated high-speed camera to record eye movements. An IMU (inertial measurement unit) is also incorporated, which records the head movements.
- This high-tech apparatus is connected to the computer with appropriate software.
- A stationary object is fixed to the wall, and the patient is asked to focus on it. The first calibration is done.
- The examiner manipulates the patient's head by quick, precise movements, usually 15 degrees to either side of the line of the patient's focus on the stationary object.

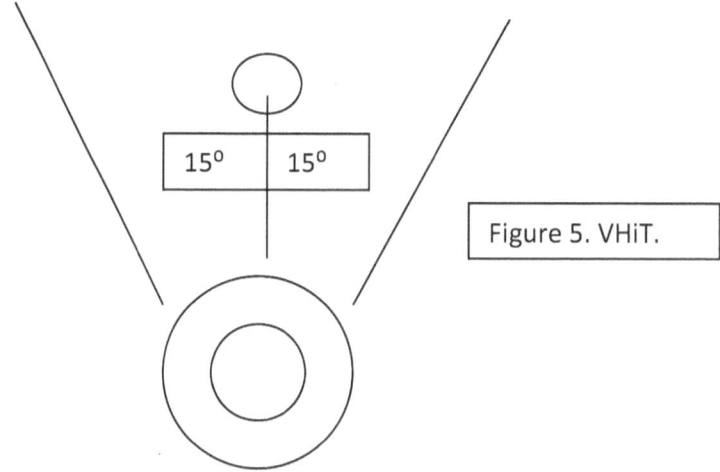

Figure 5. VHiT.

- 20 Manipulations are done on each side. The head is moved quickly to one side and then brought gently back in neutral position.
- Canals are tested as follows.
    1. Lateral (Horizontal) Canal. Moving the head in the horizontal plane.
    2. LARP (Left Anterior and Right Posterior). Both canals are oriented in the same plane, and so are RALP.

       Turn the patient's head 30–40 degrees to the right and instruct the patient that at all times, he should be looking at the fixation spot. Manipulations are now done in forward and backwards directions. They are done the same as above, repeating 20 times with 15 degrees on either side of point of focus. Forward movement will test the left anterior canal, and backwards movement will test the right posterior canal.
    3. RALP (Right Anterior and Left Posterior)

       Now turn the patient's head 30–40 degrees left and perform the test. Forward movements will now measure

the right anterior canal, and backwards will give a tracing of the left posterior canal.

- The computer performs the calculations of relationship between eye and head movements. These calculations are represented as tracings.

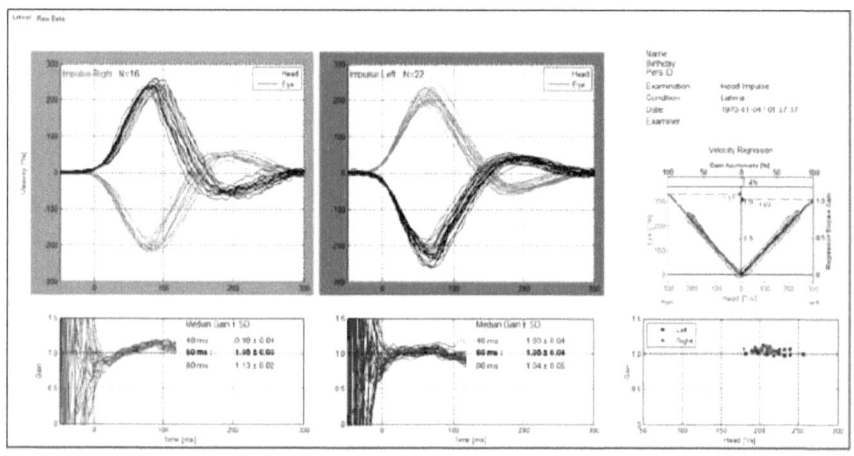

Figure 6a. Normal VOR response.

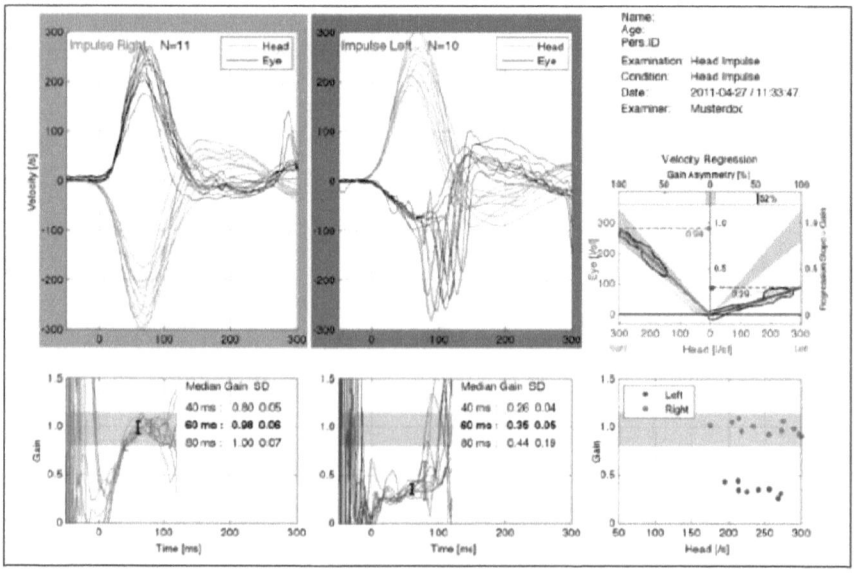

Figure 6b. Abnormal VOR response

Limitations
- Like other vestibular tests, it should be read in conjunction with clinical findings and other tests.

Computerised Dynamic Posturography (CPD)

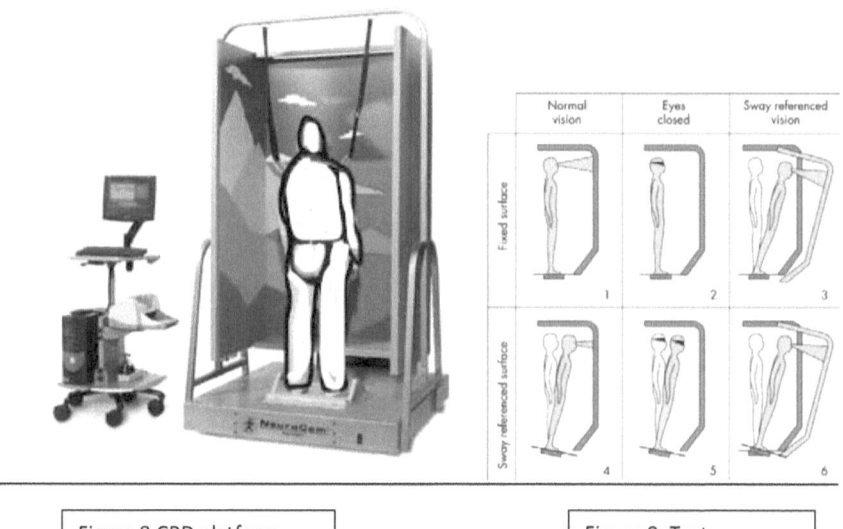

| Figure 8.CPD platform. | Figure 9. Test |

Balance function is a highly adaptive system of multiple interactive components. Computerised dynamic posturography was developed as an objective method to differentiate sensory, motor, and central adaptive functional impairment of balance.

The functional balance is a fine interaction between maintaining centre of gravity (COG) above base of support in static or dynamic situations. Base of support is area of contact between feet and the surface. Strategies to acquire the balance control will be determined by the stability or nature of the base of support (e.g., firm, mobile, rough, or smooth) because these will alter the area of contact with feet. Sensory deficits will have same effect as well.

We resist falling by constantly altering our COG relative to base of support. In cases where there are excessive movements of base, we step forward or backwards. A sudden change in base of support may cause stumbling.

Three strategies are involved during the movements.

Ankle Strategy

When the base is firm and COG movements are slow. Rotation of body takes place about the ankle joint as rigid mass.

Hip Strategy

When movements of the trunk are rapid or the base of support is unpredictable, large movements at the hip are necessary.

Step Strategy

With a very large shift in the body position or excessive movements of the base of support, a step is required to widen the base of support.

Traditional diagnostic tests (e.g., VNG) are employed to localise the pathology. CPD is a performance test. It will determine the patient's functional limitation to perform certain task.

CPD objectively assesses these limitations. It can highlight the nature of disability and help in appropriately customizing the most efficient methods in vestibular rehabilitation. CDP can be used as a tool to carry out vestibular rehabilitation by applying functional tasks to the patient in a safe and controlled environment.

Method

Equipment called an Equitest is used. It has a moving platform with a movable visual screen.

The patient is put in a harness to prevent falling and is asked to stand still on the platform with eyes open and close.

The test protocol includes:

1. Sensory organization test (SOT)
2. Motor control test (MCT)
3. Adaptation test

1. Sensory Organization Test (SOT)
   - To perform SOT somatosensory (support surface) and/ or visual input is selectively disrupted and then patient's ability to maintain the balance is measured.
   - It is performed in six different conditions.

Conditions	Vision	Base of Support	Visual Field
1	Eyes Open	Stable	Stable
2	Eyes Close	Stable	Stable
3	Eyes Open	Stable	Sway
4	Eyes Open	Sway	Stable
5	Eyes Closed	Sway	Stable
6	Eyes Open	Sway	Sway

- Each condition is tested three times for reliable results.
- Analysis is done by computer, which compares each condition to the stored data obtained from age-matched, normal individuals.
- SOT (sensory organization test) has three components:
  - Somato Sensory

- Visual: Condition 4 with Condition 1. In patients who destabilise with unpredictable base of support; this means visual input is impaired.

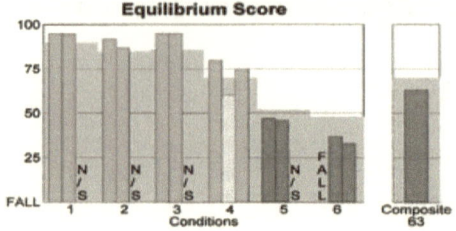

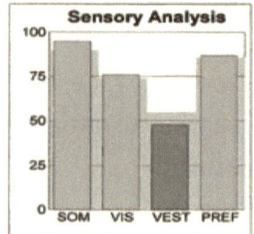
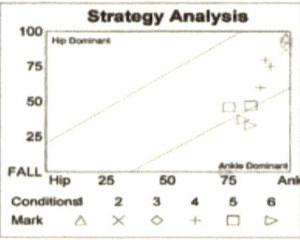
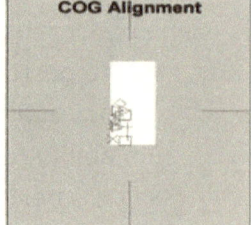

Figure 10.

- Vestibular: Condition 5 with Condition 2. Decrease in the ratio will indicate that the patient is unable to use vestibular input with an unstable base of support.
- Vision Preference: Sum of Conditions 3and6 with Sum of Conditions 2and5. Reduced ratio will indicate an inability to maintain balance by moving visual fields.

o Strategy Analysis
  - It the measure of ankle and hip movements in relation to above six conditions presented to patients.

- Conditions (represented by symbols) falling in the lower right column (for ankle) or upper left column (for hip) will indicate abnormalities.

  o COG Analysis
    - It measures the patient's response in relation to base of support.
    - All six conditions should not fall out of the central box.

2. Motor Control test (MCT)
   - Automatic reaction of the body is measured to restore the balance in response to sudden,unexpected forward or backwards displacement of base of support.
   - Results are noted by delay in latency and shifting of the weight on each leg.

3. Adaptation Test
   - It is the measure of the body's ability to suppress the automatic response to sudden change in the base of support and visual sensations.
   - It exposes the patient to toes up and toes down sequences when sudden stimuli are initiated to prevent fall.
   - Amplitude of movements is noted. Patients with balance issues will fall because they are unable to adapt.

Posturography should be read in conjunction with findings on all other tests, history, and clinical examination.

Setting up a Balance Clinic

Balance disorders are unique. Their clinical presentation can be from simple to very complicated. In a large number of cases, they are multifactorial in origin. About 45 per cent of all population above the age of forty-five will have some form of balance issue. This may be vestibular or non-vestibular in origin. The presentation of patient in the majority of cases is varied. One of the major factors in long-term chronic sufferers is lack of explanation of their symptoms and planned management. This gives rise to anxiety and can lead to depression. Vestibular symptoms in these situations further deteriorate, typically spiralling into a vicious cycle from which the patients find it difficult to get out. They lose the confidence within themselves and lose trust in the treating physician.

Ideally for these patients, a pathway with a multidisciplinary approach should be approached. Giving the patient ample time in the clinic to discuss his issue cannot be stressed enough. In one study, the measure of QoL (Quality of Life) index showed that sufferers of Ménière's scored between Alzheimer's, AIDS, and a cancer patient six weeks before death. This is really significant. One should keep that in mind when consulting the patient in the clinic. A listening ear is so important for these patients that in many cases, it becomes part of therapy in itself.

In this day and age with pressures on the healthcare system, patients with balance disorders cannot be appropriately assessed within the framework of a routine clinic. A separate arrangement and setup is recommended to evaluate these patients. Detailed evaluation and assessment with discussion, amongst other disciples, give immense confidence to patient. Giving them a diagnosis, explanation, and management plan boosts their trust, elevates them psychologically and emotionally, and gives them a different perspective to theirproblem. This is where a relationship of trust startsbetween the physician and the patient, which is so important in management.

How to Establish Referral Base

Education of the primary care and other disciples is the key. A primary care physician has significant restraints with time and finances. They may have done their best to control patient's symptoms, but due to nature and complexity of balance issues, it could easily become a losing battle. In this scenario, availability of a service which can help almost 45 per cent of their patients above forty-five years of age, and even more in elderly group, will be hugely beneficial.

It is important to establish a workable relationship or a pathway with other colleagues within the ENT department and other specialties (e.g.,neurology, medical elderly). This can be done by regular meetings and the presentations about the importance of issue. This gives them a route or pathway to refer patients who can be dealt more efficiently in a different setting.

Clinic Setup

The most important factor in a balance setup is availability of an enthusiastic physiotherapist who is trained in dealing with balance issues. Training usually will not pose a huge issue. There is certainly a sharp learning curve, but once that is achieved, the confidence to treat the patient increases very quickly. Initially a visit and possible observership in an established balance centre will be of huge value. This will be true for both the physician and physiotherapist.

A good working relationship with the audiology department cannot be stressed more. It will be an advantage to have dedicated audiologist working for a balance setup. The nature of this disorder is such that one will need friends almost everywhere (e.g., neurology, cardiology, psychiatry).

It will be important to set some basic rules for clinics. For example:

- A one-stop clinic with a multidisciplinary setup will be ideal. It is a real uphill task due to a host of logistic and financial factors.
- However, it will be most useful to establish a close liaison with audiology, neurology, and physiotherapy.
- Setting up consultation time is very important. These patients cannot be assessed in five- to ten-minutes time slots. Please remember these patients may have been suffering for a very long time, may have seen many different disciples, and may have had a variety of explanations and diagnoses of their symptoms. It is important to extract accurate history as much as you can. Patients should be made comfortable, andevery effort is spent to concentrate on patients. This will go a long way in establishing a healthy relationship with patients.
- It is important to send or hand over the balance questionnaire to patients before the first consultation. It will be very useful to acquire a good history of symptoms and functional abilities of the patients.

Equipment for Clinic

One does not need a lot of equipment or fancy gadgets to run a successful balance clinic.

- A basic ENT trolley equipped for routine ENT examination will be required.

- A Snellen's chart andopthalmoscope for cranial nerve examination will be useful.
- A couch with adjustable head end or tilt mechanism will be needed.
- A piece of two-inch-thick foam (2×2 feet) will be helpful.

    These will be more than enough to run a balance clinic. There are other specialised equipment available, such as:
    - Frenzel glasses (removes visual fixation when testing for nystagmus)
    - VNG if available

The most important part of setting up a dedicated balance clinic is the time one can give to patients to understand their day-to-day sufferings, and to find and innovative methods to help them. Quite frequently there may not be one single diagnosis in these patients, but extracting out what one can help with in these patients will be very satisfying to them.

Balance Disorders

Balance disorders can be categorised as follows.

- Episodic
    - Vestibular migraine
    - Ménière's
    - BPPV
    - Other causes: PLF, SC dehiscence, cardiovascular(postural hypotension, arrythmias), episodic ataxia
- Chronic Imbalance
    - Vestibulopathies
    - Persistent postural perceptual dizziness (PPPD)
    - Mal debarquement syndrome (MdDS)
    - Neurological (peripheral neuropathies, Parkinson's, epilepsy)
    - Multisensory balance disorders (usually in elderly)
    - Psychological
    - Musculoskeletal
    - Visual disturbance
    - Drug related

Balance disorders can present as acute vestibulopathy and chronic imbalance problems. Common episodic balance problems are discussed elsewhere.

Acute Vestibulopathies

Condition	Presentation	Duration	Associated Factors	Treatment
Vestibular Neuronitis	Single event acute dizziness/ imbalance	Days	None	Symptomatic
Labrynthitis	Single event acute dizziness/ imbalance	Days	Hearing loss	Symptomatic steroid oral/ intratympanic
Ménière's	Episodic true vertigo	Hours	Tinnitus, SN hearing loss (fluctuant)	Symptomatic in acute episode then diet, medications, ITS, etc.
Vestibular Migraine	Acute vertigo/ imbalance, photophobia, phonophobia, rarely tinnitus, hearing loss	Minutes/ hours to days	Headaches, aura, migraine trigger factors	Treatment of migraine (i.e., avoid trigger factors), medical therapy, VRT
BPPV	True vertigo with head movement	Seconds	Can be imbalance	Canalith repositioning manoeuvre
Post Fossa lesions	Sudden Vertigo, Neurological Symptoms and Signs	Minutes(TIA), but can be days	Central/ ocular signs	As per stroke protocol
Perilymph Fistula	Sudden attacks of dizziness several times a day. History of injury/ ontological surgery	Seconds	Fluctuant hearing loss	Surgical

Superior Semicircular Canal Dehescence	Imbalance, ocillopsia, autophony	Seconds	Fluctuant hearing loss. pressure	Surgical

Chronic Vestibulopathies

➢ Persistent Postural Perceptual Dizziness (PPPD)
  o This is a newly recognised syndrome which almost constitutes 10–15 per cent of dizzy clinic patients. It was first described in 1986 by a neurologist as phobic postural dizziness (PPD). Initially it was thought to be strongly linked with underlying psychological disorders of patient. Further studies, however, revealed that it is a neuro-otological condition which is more common in certain types of psychiatric conditions (e.g., obsessive compulsive personality or mild anxiety). This condition was increasing and recognised for further studies, and in 2017, WHO included PPPD in its list of International Classification of Diseases.

Presentation
  o The primary symptoms of PPPD are a persistent sensation of rocking or swaying unsteadiness lasting three months or more. This will be with the background of underlying previous chronic balance issues.
  o Symptoms are typically worse with:
    1. Upright posture (standing or sitting upright; may disappear on lying)
    2. Head or body motion
    3. Exposure to motion-rich environments.

- Patients avoid situations which make their symptoms worse,such as visually challenged places (e.g., busy supermarket). The patients become afraid that something terrible may happen. This is a physical condition that may end up having psychological effects.

- Trigger Factors

    There are a number of trigger factors which may start this condition.

    1. Peripheral or central balance disorders (e.g.,vestibular neuronitis, Ménière's, BPPV, stroke)
    2. Vestibular migraine
    3. Mild traumatic brain injury
    4. nability to compensate fully after initial vestibular insult.
    5. Anxieties may predispose to this condition. Almost 60 per cent of PPPD patients have anxieties.

- Diagnosis
    - It is mainly clinical. Typically, all the tests are normal. The tests are not done to diagnose this condition; rather, they are performed to rule out other co-morbidities.
- Treatment
    - Counselling: It is important to these patients that someone spends time with them to explain the diagnosis and pathways of treatment.
    - Medical: Selective serotonin reuptake inhibitors (SSRI) like Citalopram and Fluoxatine have been tried with some success.
    - Vestibular Rehabilitation: This goes a long way and is perhaps the most effective way of treatment.

> ➢ Mal De'Barquement Syndrome
>> ○ Mal de'barquement literally means sickness of disembarkment. It is the illusion of movements.
>> ○ This can affect some people after travelling in a boat or ship, but it can follow airplane travel, usually after long-haul flights.
>> ○ Most people experience this illusion of movements immediately after the event. It resolves within short period of time, usually within twenty-four hours. If it lasts more than one month, then it is defined as Mel de'barquement syndrome. It is not known why it becomes persistent in some people.
>
>> ○ Presentation
>
>>> ○ The patient feels rocking or swaying all the time. There is no true vertigo. It is usually precipitated by sea travel but can be after a long-haul flight.
>>> ○ Symptoms improve with continuous motions such as driving, and they get worse when patients are motionless. Stress and fatigue worsen the symptoms.
>>> ○ It can be a disabling condition in some people and can affect quality of life.
>>> ○ This condition resolves spontaneously within one year in the majority of people.
>
>> ○ Diagnosis
>
>>> ○ There is no specific investigation of this condition. It is diagnosed on clinical grounds.

o   Treatment

    o   There is no specific treatment for this condition. In early stages, control of symptoms can be achieved by short-term use of Prochlorperazine or standard travel sickness medications. Vestibular rehabilitation may be useful in persistently symptomatic patients.

Management Of Ménière's Disease

❦

Ménière's disease, also called idiopathic endolymphatic hydrops, is a disorder of the inner ear. Although the cause is unknown, it probably results from an abnormality in the fluids of the inner ear. Ménière's disease is one of the most common causes of dizziness originating in the inner ear. The incidence of Ménière's in general population is one in one thousand. As much as 30–50 per cent can be bilateral, which is a relatively high proportion. It is commoner in females. It can be seen in all age groups but has a higher prevalence in the age group of thirty to forty.

Aetiology

The commonest cause is idiopathic in nature, and in this case it is termed as Ménière's disease. If the cause is known, it is called Ménière's syndrome. Some common reasons are post-infection (CSOM, labrynthitis, syphilis),trauma (acoustic trauma, fracture temporal bone, surgical trauma),or autoimmune disorders (Cogan disease,visual difficulties, hearing loss,dizziness).

Pathophysiology

It is the dysfunction of the endolymphatic system where there is either inadequate absorption or excessive production of endolymph. Some theories have been put forward to support it.
- Saccin Theory
  - Blockage of the endolymphatic duct causes production of hormone called saccin. That leads to dilatation of the endolymphatic sac. Membranous labyrinth ruptures induce an attack. It repairs itself in a few hours to twenty-four. That is when the attack subsides. Recurrent rupture leads to the burned-out stage.
- Dark Cell Theory
  - Dark cells produce excessive endolymph, leading to the above cycle.

Variants of Ménière's

- Vestibular Hydrops
  - Episodic vertigo only (20 per cent will develop Ménière's)
- Cochlear Hydrops
  - Hearing loss and tinnitus only (80 per cent will develop Ménière's)
- Tumarkin Otolithic Crises
  - Sudden drop attacks without any warning; can lose consciousness
  - Possible indication of the end stage of disease
  - Affects 2 per cent of Ménière's patients
- Leromoyez syndrome (rare variant, tinnitus, HL, and aural fullness are relieved by vertigo attack instead of increasing)

Differential Diagnosis

- Vestibular migraine
- Trauma (surgical or fracture temporal bone)
- Perilymph fistula
- Acoustic neuroma
- Autoimmune inner ear disorder
- Thyroid disease
- Diabetes
- Large vestibular aqueduct syndrome

Clinical Presentation

Classic Ménière's presentation is a combination of aural fullness, episodic vertigo (lasting between minutes to twenty-four hours), tinnitus, and low-frequency fluctuating sensorineural hearing loss.

There may be associated nausea and vomiting, sweating, and diarrhoea. It should be noted that migraine-associated vertigo (MAV) prevalence is 40–50 per cent in Ménière's patients.

Clinical Staging

Staging the disease can help in assessing the clinical progression, and it makes documentation easier.

Stage 1
- Classical symptoms. The patient will have normal hearing between attacks.

Stage 2
- The patient will establish permanent hearing loss (typically low frequency).

Stage 3
- Hearing loss becomes worse, with constant disequilibrium rather than episodic vertigo. This is also known as the 'burned out' stage.

Assessment

- Full Neuro-otologic Examination. Commonly normal in early stages. However, it may show signs of vestibular failure and, in some cases, positive findings of concurrent issues (e.g., BPPV).
- Pure Tone Audiometry. Classically shows fluctuating low-frequency sensorineural hearing loss. This is almost the diagnostic criterion for the disease. In late stages, the hearing loss becomes irreversible and constant.
- MRI to rule out Acoustic Neuroma.
- Lab Investigations: FBC, PV, BCP, BG. In case of B/L autoimmune profile, syphilis serology.
- VNG/Calorics (May be normal)
- VHiT (Video Head Impulse Test). This test is gaining popularity. It can be done to assess concurrent vestibular failure.
- Electrocochleography. Not commonly done. Can be very painful to perform. It is specific but not sensitive.

Diagnosis of Ménière's is primarily clinical. Good history supported by serial audiograms showing fluctuant SN hearing loss is diagnostic. The entire battery of tests outlined above will help to rule out other causes with similar clinical presentation and can also be useful in long-term management of the disease.

Management

Natural history of this problem is quite variable. Many patients will remain mildly affected. However, in its severe form Ménière's can be a significantly disabling entity. In one study of the quality of life index, it was shown that a patient with Ménière's scored the same as patient with cancersix weeks before death. This highlights the severity of the illness.

- First Line of Management

  It is very important to evaluate the patient's general psychological make-up, levels of stress, anxiety, work environment, and dietary habits in the first interview. This will form the basis of counselling, which may be needed in very early stages of the disease.

  Before starting any medical treatment, a detailed counselling session is given to the patient regarding:

  1. Lifestyle change, which will include dietary habits. Provision of a full dietary sheet will be ideal; specifically,a decrease in caffeine (coffee, tea, colas) and salt intake is of paramount importance.
  2. Reassurance, explanation of the disease process, and natural history of the disease.
  3. Psychological evaluation and the therapy, if indicated.

- Medical Therapy

  1. Commonly Used Drugs
     - For the Acute Phase: Vestibular sedatives (Cinnazine) andantiemetics (Stemetil, Buccastem) are used for a short period.

- Long-term Medical Therapy:
  - Betahistine (SERC) 16mg TDS. In severe cases, a higher dose of 24mg TDS is recommended for a few months. Recent studies have shown that SERC has no role in the control of Ménière's. However, it is used widely. It is a low-risk treatment, and many patients swear by it.
  - Diuretics, usually Bendrofluazide 2.5mg OD. There is variable success with this treatment. Side effects, especially of lowering K+ levels, should be kept in mind.

  - Vestibular Physiotherapy: It has its own role in the management of Ménière's. In general, classical Ménière's, with its fluctuant presentation, will not be suitable for vestibular rehab. However, in certain situations(e.g., presence of concurrent balance issues,vestibular failure, or BPPV), it can be employed very successfully in treatment.
2. In a large majority of cases, these measures will suffice. A satisfactory and long-term control of the disease can be achieved for most patients.
3. If the symptoms fail to settle, then therapy will be stepped up.

- Second Line of Management
  - There are a number of options available to step up a patient's treatment. The choice of these varies between different physicians

and their experience. Controversies also exist amongst the methods and techniques employed. However, recent studies have shown very encouraging results of intratympanic steroids, and it is becoming increasingly popular.

This form of treatment comes more in the domain of super specialization of balance disorders.

Use of Intratympanic Medical Therapy

There is a long history of intratympanic use of different medications.

- Barany used Lignocain for Tinnitus in 1935
- Beur used urea for glue ears in 1971
- Bryne used steroids for facial paralysis in 1973
- Shucknecht was the first to propose amino glycoside for Ménière's in 1948
- Silverstein used steroids for sensorineural hearing loss in 1996
- Itoh used steroids for Ménière's in 1991

1. Intratympanic Steroids
   - Complete resolution of vertiginous symptoms may be expected with the use of intratympanic steroids. They are also very effective in controlling the acute flare-up of the disease.
   - It has gained popularity due to excellent results, very few complications, and ease of use.
   - There are almost no contraindications as opposed to the use of oral steroids.

- Mechanism of Action
    1. Different theories have been postulated to describe the possible mechanism of action.
        - It is thought that steroids reduce the inflammation, however there is no evidence base to follow.
        - Intratympanic use of medications bypasses the blood labyrinthine barrier. It is thought that intratympanic steroids are 260 times more effective than oral steroids in Ménière's.
        - The drug mainly enters inner ear through RWM but can be through the oval window and cochlear bone.
- Indications

The decision to use ITS in Ménière's is mostly experience based. Recent studies advocate the use of ITS very early in the course of disease. It can be used in the following situations.

1. Recent studies have shown that it can be used as a first-line treatment of Ménière's. The results have been very encouraging.
2. Acute, non-resolving symptoms.
3. Other issues limiting aggressive or full medical therapy (e.g., age-related issues or compliance of drugs).

- Delivery of Intratympanic Steroids

1. There not any standard protocol for dose, frequency, concentration, or type for intratympanic steroids
2. The majority of people use Dexamethasone or Mythyle prednisolone. Steroid gels have been tried. The use of gel is still under research. They

can be left in middle ear for a longer period to improve the efficacy. New research has shown Methyleprednisolone has better long-term results.

3. The dose of Dexamethasone is 3.3mg/mL, and Methyleprednisolone is 40mg/mL.
4. There are a number of different delivery methods that have been described.
   - Delivery with fine bore needle (29G spinal needle).
   - After Myringotomy: Done in the anteriosuperior quadrant (not a favoured method).
   - After placing Grommet:
     - Grommet makes it easier to institute repeated application.
     - Practical delivery of medication is limited because it easily gets airlocked during the process of intratympanic injection.
     - Medication can be introduced through Grommet by either:
       - Fine needle
       - Steroid eardrops
       - Micro wick

- Method
  1. Preferred method is with fine bore needle (29G spinal needle) using 1mL (insulin syringe), 2mL, or 5mLsyringes.
  2. It is an outpatient procedure.

- Anaesthesia
  1. Usually local anaesthetic, but can be done without any anaesthetic.
     - EMLA cream
       - It is very effective.

- Common due to ease of use.
- Always introduce under microscope to make sure EMLA is in contact with tympanic membrane.
- Leave it for 45–60 minutes.

- Phenol

  Very effective and quick, but there is a high risk of perforation.

- Delivery

  - Size 29G spinal needle is ideal because risk of perforation is small, and backspill of medication is very little.
  - Up to 1.0–1.5mL can be delivered in middle ear in posterio-inferior quadrant,so the delivery will be aimed as close to round window as possible.

- Postinjection Instructions to patient
  - Lie on good ear for 15–20minutes.
  - Do not swallow.
  - Some dizziness is expected after injection.
  - Blocked sensation in the injected ear is to be expected.

- Complications
  - a. In some patients, it can be very painful.
  - b. Tympanic membrane perforation. More common if phenol is used as local anaesthetic agent.
  - c. Non-resolution of the symptoms.

    d. Patient will have blocked sensation and possibly mild conductive hearing loss for few days after injection.

Intratympanic Gentamicin Injection

- This is also known as chemical labyrinthectomy.
- Very effective with carefully selected patients. Success rate can be as good as 80–90 per cent.
- Patient should be counselled fully regarding the facts listed below.
  1. Potential hearing loss. Can be up to 25–30db in as much as 40–50 per cent of cases. It can be lower in some cases. High frequency loss is common.
  2. Dead ear (5 per cent).
  3. Expected dizziness for up to six weeks before compensation takes place.
  4. Non-resolution of tinnitus and existing hearing loss.
  5. Recurrence of symptoms
     - Early: In cases of Gentamicin failure (commonly due to Gentamicin resistance and round window adhesions).
     - Late: In cases of Ménière's involving the other side (30–50 per cent).

- Selection of Patients for Chemical Labyrinthectomy
  1. This modality of treatment comes after all avenues of conservative treatment have failed.

2. Patient should be counselled comprehensively about all aspects of the treatment and outcome as outlined above.
3. It is imperative to do a pre-injection audiogram.
4. Decision should be taken after mutual agreement.
5. It should be regarded as a major change in the direction of the treatment.

- Indications
  - Non-resolving unilateral Ménière's after full medical treatment.
  - Otolithic crises.

- Method
  - No standard protocol. Anaesthetics, procedures, and delivery methods are about same as described above for intratympanic steroid injections.
  - In cases of failure of injection therapy, a more intrusive method of tympanotomy and leaving Gentamicin-soaked gelfoam over round window is used.
  - Some centres employ this method as routine because it is claimed that incidence of hearing loss is less due to the fact that amount of Gentamicin used is less and applied directly to round window.
  - It is also the method of choice where adhesions in the round window niche are suspected.

- Dose
  - 0.5 mL of 40mg/mL solution = 20mg of Gentamicin without dilution is used.
  - 2–3 injections at 4 weekly intervals.

- Pre-injection and Postinjection Care
  - Imperative to do pre-injection audiogram before each application.
  - It will be ideal if facility to check 16K and 32K frequencies are available.
  - Ask patient to lie on good ear for 20 minutes.
  - Instruct patient to not swallow.
  - Patient is not allowed to drive immediately after the treatment.
  - Patient is expected to recover in roughly 6–8 weeks after finishing the injection therapy.
  - In the following visits, depending on the patient's response, his medications for Ménière's can be slowly tapered off.

- Complications and Their Management
  1. 15–20 per cent of patients sustain significant hearing loss. This loss is usually is in the high frequency.
  2. Dead ear. Cross Aid hearing aid or cochlear implant.
  3. Failure to resolve symptoms.
     - This could be either complete failure with persistence of Ménière's symptoms. May be due to:
       - RWM adhesions. Alternative delivery method of tympanotomy and placement of Gentamicin-soaked gelfoam at round window after removal of adhesions.
       - Gentamicin resistance. Can be very difficult to overcome.

- Bilateral Disease.
  - In as many as 30–50 per cent of cases, bilateral disease is present, and it is very troublesome to treat. Management is day-to-day control of symptoms by medication, changing lifestyle, and psychological support (e.g., counselling can be helpful).

There are some modalities of treatment which were widely in use for a very long time. Recent studies have shown that they have very little effect on the course of the disease. I will briefly describe them.

1. Grommet Insertion
   - One of the earliest conservative surgical methods.
   - It can be done as an office procedure.
   - No rationale, but it does work 50 per cent of the time on its own.
   - These days, it's mostly used when intratympanic steroids or Gentamicin is planned to avoid repeated injections.
   - It is also used before starting therapy with a Meniett device.
2. Meniett Device
   - It is micropressure therapy. Small, portable device delivers computer-controlled, low-pressure waves via a fine catheter. This catheter is introduced through a grommet in the middle ear.
   - Not available commonly.
   - It is expensive.

- There are controversies around its efficacy due to variable results.

- Third Line of Management
  - Usually, they are surgical ablative procedures.
  - Done for patients with non-remittent, frequent, and severe attacks.

1. Endolymphatic Succuss Decompression
   - Preserves hearing
   - Success rates are about 60 per cent, however some trials have shown it failed to show superior results as compared to a sham operation

2. Osseous Labirynthectomy
   - Complete loss of hearing
   - Major surgical procedure

3. Vestibular Neurectomy
   - Major surgery
   - Risk of injury to cranial nerves.

Vestibular Migraine

A migraine is described as a primary headache disorder by the International Headache Society Classification. It is characterised by recurrent moderate to severe headaches, typically on one side of head, with associated nausea, vomiting, and sensitivity to light and sound.

It has been postulated that as much as 40 per cent patients with migraines have some vestibular issues. About 15 per cent of migraine patients present with predominant vestibular symptoms rather than headaches. Some of them can be termed as 'migraine without headaches'because there may be almost a complete absence of headache symptoms.

Almost 50 per cent of migraines remain undiagnosed because they are self-treated or misdiagnosed as sinus pains or other non-migrainous causes.

Vestibular migraines are the most common cause of recurrent vertigo.

Presentation
- Dizziness could be of any type from true vertigo to imbalance issues.
- Commonly in the 20–40 years age group.
- More common in females with a ratio of 3:1.

- Most common vestibular disorder in children and young adults.
- In children. BPPV is regarded as a variant of vestibular migraine.
- It can mimic Ménière's with attacks of true vertigo and aural symptoms, but it usually does not fulfil the criteria of Ménière's. The attacks usually last much longer (could be from minutes to weeks). The patient may continue to have problem in between episodes, and hearing loss is not progressive. It is interesting to note that there is a 40 per cent prevalence of VM in Ménière's.
- As many as 10–40 per centof patients may present with cochlear symptoms like hearing loss and tinnitus.
- Increased sensitivity to motion and sound is typical.
- Can be associated with anxiety and panic attacks.
- Stress may be an aggravating factor.
- Sometimes can present with BPPV. This has been described as associated migraine syndrome in IHS classification.

Pathophysiology
- The exact mechanism is still not completely understood, but vascular theory has long been accepted.
- It is now thought it is due to altered vascular and neural mechanism.
- Hereditary predisposition is an important factor that can give rise to abnormal discharge of neurons, especially in the brainstem area. Hence, vestibular involvement can be explained.
- It is also postulated that there is spontaneous spread of abnormal electrical discharge to cerebral cortex as well that can activate pain receptors.
- A number of factors have been described that can trigger migraines.
  o Food triggers, especially caffeine, certain dairy products, red wine, Chinese food (monosodium

glutamate), and hypoglycaemia (which can be transient).
- o Other factors like stress, lack of sleep, hormonal changes, and change in middle ear pressure.

Diagnosis
- History has a pivotal role.
  - o Presentation of symptoms is usually variable and can be vague.
  - o History sometimes can be very suggestive of Ménière's or BPPV. Fine differences should be very carefully deciphered.
  - o History of associated symptoms is important (e.g., motion sickness, sensitivity to light or sound).
  - o Previous or family history of migraine.
  - o History of associated symptoms (e.g., headaches, travel sickness, sensitivity to bright light, stress, anxiety),
- Examination
  - o Important to note patient's psychological outlook.
  - o Clinically may not be able to elicit any positive signs.
  - o Should carry out full otoneurologic examination.
- Investigations
  - o If any neurological deficit is present, then perform an MRI.
  - o Balance tests have a variable place in the assessment.
  - o Patients with a vestibular migraine usually react quite violently to the caloric test.

Treatment

Most of the patients of vestibular migraine consulting in a balance clinic are not aware of the diagnosis, or they do not think their balance issues have any relationship to migraines. Therefore it is important that they are made aware of the underlying problem andthat a management plan is discussed with them after an appropriate session of counselling.

It will be good practice to provide the patients with relevant written information to take home. It is a known fact that most patients will only be able to digest 50 per cent of the verbal information given to them.

Management of vestibular migraine will have a somewhat different approach as opposed to conventional migraine therapy. There are two aspects of VM treatment. One is therapy for migraine, and the second is addressing the associated balance issues.

Management of migraines should start with detailed explanation of the patient's condition and symptoms. More often than not, most people do not relate migrainesto balance issues. Migraines are usually thought to be a type of headache.

First Line of Management

- Lifestyle changes.
    - ○ Information about trigger factors (dietary, stress, hormonal). It will be useful to have a full list of common dietary and other triggers to hand it to patients. It is important to actively ask patients about their dietary habits, such as caffeine intake and how many meals they take in a day. (Not uncommonly, people miss meals during day for a variety of reasons. Due to fluctuation of blood sugar levels, it may turn out to be a trigger factor.)
    - ○ Work-related issues (e.g., stress, workplace layout). Some people find it difficult to work in open-plan spaces or with certain lighting arrangements and computer screens. These are all small background

details but may have quite a large impact on patients without their awareness.

- o Keeping a diary of headaches and related balance problems may be useful for patient and clinician for long-term management.
- o These all should be discussed with the patients, and strategies should be outlined to address these issues in their personal lives and working environment. Sometimes patients need a doctor's help to support them by informing and directing their employers to optimise work conditions for them.
- o It is a possibility that patients may not have shared these details with any therapist before, and highlighting them will increase their confidence. This may help to alleviate anxiety and will lead to better outcome of treatment.

Second Line of Management

Medical Therapy

There is not any one specific medication available to treat migraines. The medical treatment can vary in every patient. It is important to find out or at least narrow down the trigger factor causing the primary issue.

The medical therapy can be divided into the treatment of acute attack and preventive therapy.

Acute Medical Therapyfor Migraine

There are a variety of medications and combinations pills available. They are used according to the individual patient's response.

- They could be as simple as paracetamol, aspirin, NSAIDs, or combined pills like:

- o Migraleve (paracetamol and codeine)
- o ParamaMax (paracetamol and metaclopromide)
- o MigraMax (Aspirin and metaclopromide)
- Antiemetics
- Migraine Specific:
  - o Triptans (e.g., Sumatrypitan, Imigran)
    - Mechanismof Action: They are serotonin (5 HT1) agonist. They act by constricting the blood vessels in the head and block transmission of pain to skin and face.
    - Should not be used in patients with ischemic heart disease.
    - Side Effects: Tingling,heaviness, tightness in throat or chest.
  - o Others, like Ergot alkaloids, are rarely used due to side effects and tolerance issues.

Preventive Medical Therapy:

They are important in long-term management of patients. Usually they are started if the attacks are frequent. It could take up to three months for prophylactic treatment to take effect.

- Beta Blockers (Propranolol)
  - o Mechanism of Action: Reduce dilatation of blood vessels.
  - o It is a useful first-line prevention, especially in patients with anxiety.
  - o Should not be used in patients with asthma or cardiac issues like heart block.
  - o Side Effects: GI upset, bradycardia, fatigue,aggravated dizziness.
  - o Dose: Can be started in a low dose like 10mg Od and then gradually built up. Prophylactic dose is 40mg BD or slow release preparations.

- Tricyclic Antidepressents (Amitryptaline, Nortryptaline)
  - Mechanism of Action: Block re-uptake of 5HT and norepinephrine.
  - Should not be used in patients with epilepsy and cardiac disease.
  - Side Effects: Dry mouth, drowsiness, blurred vision.
  - Dose: Initially given in small doses (10mg) at night and then gradually built up to 50 mg at night or 25mg BD. This is to reduce side effects and to increase the tolerance.
- Anti-Serotogenic (Anti 5HT) Pizotifen
  - Mechanismof Action: Serotonin antagonist and antihistamine.
  - Caution in pregnancy orrenal impairment.
  - Side Effects: Weight gain, drowsiness.
  - Dose: To start in low dose (500mcg) at night with max up to 3mg.
- Anticonvulsants (Topiramate)
  - Mechanismof Action: It is not clear for migraines. It may reduce capacity of nerves to transmit the pain.
  - Contraindicated in breastfeeding.
  - Side effects: Abdominal pain, nausea, weight loss,impaired concentration and memory.
  - Dose: 25mg OD at night for one week, then increasing in steps of 25mg at weekly intervals. Max up to 50–100mg/day.

There are other medications as well, like calcium channel blockers or Angiotensin II blockers. It will be appropriate to involve a neurologist in patients with long-term management of migraine. Balance issues are very difficult to address without optimal control of migraine, especially in the presence of concurrent Ménière's disease, anxiety, and other vestibular disorders.

Vestibular Rehabilitation in VM

As discussed earlier, the treatment of migraine has two arms, conventional migraine therapy and vestibular rehab. Addressing the balance issue in these patients at an early stage can prove to be very beneficial. In most cases, simply improving their VOR deficit works very well because most of these patients are visually oversensitised.

In general, thevestibular migraine is now recognised as one of the most common causes of balance disorders. It may be difficult to diagnose due to its varied and atypical presentation. Its early recognition and treatment can make an immense difference in these patients.

Benign Paroxysmal Positional Vertigo (BPPV)

∽

BPPV is the most common cause of vertigo. Almost 25% of the patients in the balance clinic are referred with this disorder. In fact the real incidence could be much higher as this condition is self limiting and many patients recover spontaneously. There is higher prevalence in elderly patients. Women are affected twice as much. BPPV is the most successfully treatable balance disorder.

Aetiology
- Idiopathic (most Common)
- Head injury (or even bang on the head)
- Infections
- Due to pre-existing labyrinthine condition e.g. Ménière's, Vestibular neuronitis, vestibular Migraine
- Age related (Common in elderly)

Pathophysiology

The most accepted theory is migration of otoconia from the utricle to the semicircular canal. Otoconia are the calcium carbonate crystals which are present in otolith organs. Otoconia from the saccule are unable to make their way into the canal system. They are dislodged from their original position in the utricle and most commonly migrate to the posterior semicircular canal (PC). This may be due to the fact that the posterior canal is most gravity dependent in neutral position. The presence of otoliths modifies the mechanism of stimulation of the canal from angular detector to linear detector. As a result of that, every time the head is moved, there is abnormal input in the canal leading to a brief episode of vertigo. Typically, turning in bed, looking up (e.g., top of curtain) or looking down (tying shoelaces) will produce the symptoms.

Otoconia can migrate to other canals in the vestibular system, leading to variants of BPPV. These variants can be:
- Lateral canalithiasis (LC)
- Anterior/superior canalithiasis
- Cupulolthiasis. Stuck to cupula. Commonly in lateral canal.
- Multicanal pattern

The presentation and treatment of these variants will have some differences. It is important to recognise these differences; otherwise, it can result in the failure of a patient's response to the treatment.

Presentation

The classic attack of BPPV is described as onset of true vertigo, which can be triggered by lying in bed and turning the head to the affected side, looking up (e.g., hanging the washing), or looking down (e.g., tying shoelaces).

It will usually last 20–30 seconds but no longer than a minute. However, patients may feel off balance, lasting from hours to days.

Presentation of variants can differ slightly.
- In LC, nystagmus may be horizontal, not torsional, and can be on both sides. However, it will be stronger on the affected side.
- In cupulolithiasis, nystagmus will last as long as head is kept in the lateral position, and latency can increase.

- Frequent recurrence of symptoms.
- Sometimes failure of the conventional treatment (like Epleys) may indicate presence of variant form.

Differential Diagnosis

- Migrainous vertigo: History of migraine; symptoms can be excessively prolonged. Any type of nystagmus can be expected.
- Central positional vertigo: Variable duration of attacks, which are typically prolonged with variable provoking factors. Nystagmus can be any type. There may be cerebellar or brainstem signs.
- Positional alcohol vertigo: History of alcohol abuse.
- Perilymph fistula: Typical History. Audiological signs and symptoms. Increase in vertigo with coughing, sneezing, or with valsalva may be present.
- Cervical vertigo: History of neck injury, whiplash injury. May be other neurological features. Typical association with neck movements.

Clinical Examination

In a classical case, the history is very typical. However, the diagnosis is made by eliciting typical positional nystagmus in Dix Hallpike Test.

Dix Hallpike Test

This is pathognomonic for BPPV. It is recommended to perform this test in all balance patients because it is possible that patients with BPPV sometimes become so adaptive that they successfully develop strategies to avoid becoming dizzy. It is performed as follows.

- Ask the patient to sit on the couch upright with head turned 45 degrees to one side.

- Instruct the patient to keep the eyes open and lie swiftly so that head is at 30 degrees to the body. Stay in the position up to 30seconds. Then sit the patient upright again and perform the test on the other side.
- Watch for nystagmus. In a typical PC-BPPV, it will be torsional geotropic nystagmus (fast component towards ground). Features to be noted in nystagmus are:
    - Latency: Normal is 2–6seconds. (May be absent in Lat Canalithiasis or increased in Cupulolithiasis.)
    - Duration: normal is less than 30 seconds. (In Cupulolithiasis, it will last as long as head is tilted.)
    - Fatigability: Nystagmus will not be reproducible with successive tests.
    - When patient is returned to sitting position, a transient nystagmus in the opposite direction may be noted.

Investigations

It will depend on the history and the clinical assessment.
- In a majority of patients with typical BPPV presentation, no investigation is required.
- Audiometric evaluation is done in cases where there is associated hearing loss.
- A patient who presents with excessive dizziness or vomiting following Dix Hallpike or unexplained neurological presentation should have an MRI.

Treatment

Repositioning manoeuvres are the treatment of choice. Most common is the Epley manoeuvre. Others that can be used are Semont's manoeuvre and a modified Epley and Brandt-Daroff (as home treatment). For variants like lateral canalithiasis, log roll (also called barbecue roll) can be used.

Different ways have been described to modify the Epley (e.g.,applying a vibrator on the mastoid bone of the affected side while doing Epley). Keeping the head slightly up rather than at 30 degrees with the body is another way.

Semont's manoeuvre can be attempted in recurrent cases when Epley has failed.

Restrict movements of head for a few days post-Epley and continue the modified Epley manoeuvre at home till symptoms disappear. There have been limited studies into it, but no significant difference has been noted.

Success rate of treating the BPPV with these manoeuvres is almost 80–90 per cent, and for this reason BPPV is considered as the most successfully treatable cause of balance problems.

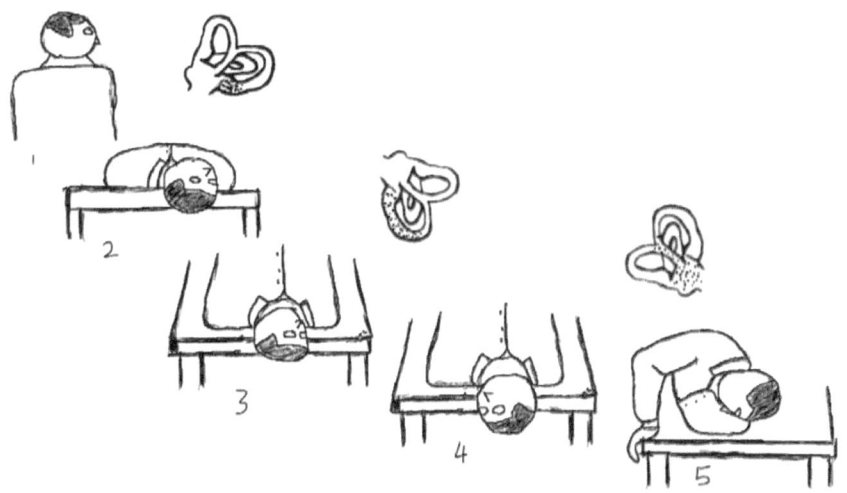

Fig Figure 11. Epley manoeuvre.

Epley Repositioning Method
- Sit patient with head turned 45 degrees to affected side.
- Quickly lie the patient down so head is at a 30-degrees angle to the body. (as in Hallpike). Maintain position for 30seconds.

- Rotate head to opposite side almost 180 degrees, maintaining the dependent position for 30seconds.
- Further rotate the head by **90** degrees so face is obliquely downwards, or ask the patient to put his nose against the couch. Leave in this position for 60seconds.
- Ask the patient to swing the legs and sit up on couch.

Post-Epley instruction to patients is also useful. These are as follows.
- Sleep propped up for at least two nights.
- Do not sleep on affected side for two nights.
- Cancel appointment with dentist or hairdresser for one week

A few patients feel off balance or fuzzy head up to a week after Epley. In our practice, we ask the patient to start Brandt-Daroff exercises (home treatment) if the symptoms do not fully subside.

The Brandt-Daroff exercise is the same as Semont's manoeuvre with a slight change. It is done by the patients themselves. It should be done five times for at least twice daily until the patient's symptoms disappear.

Treatment and Presentation of Variants of BPPV

These may present with few subtle differences from classical Posterior canal symptoms. It is important to recognise these differences as it can be challenging to treat they are not recognised.

Lateral Canalithiasis
- It should be suspected in cases which present with longstanding BPPV.
- Horizontal nystagmus on either side. (In PC-BPPV it is geotropic and torsional).

- There may not be any latency in the nystagmus (in PC-BPPV it is 2–6 seconds).
- Treatment will start with Appiani/Goufani manoeuvre but log roll can be useful.

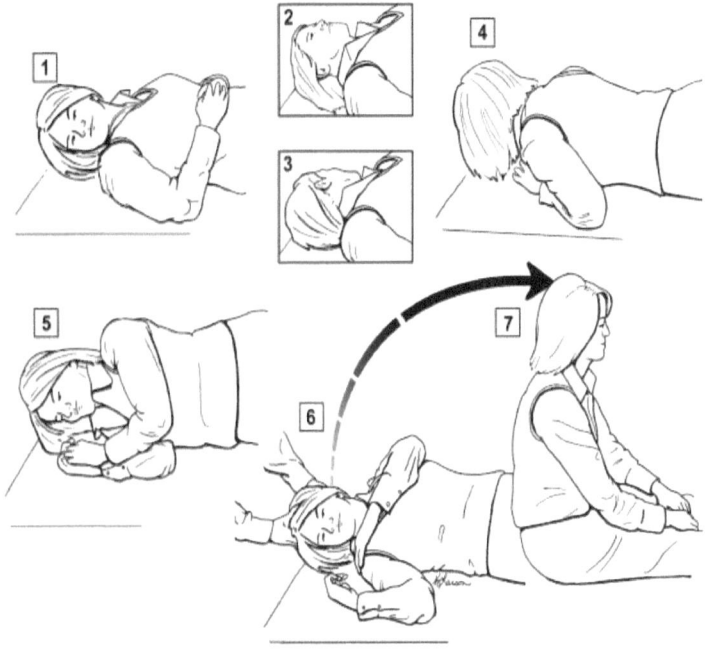

Figure 12. Log roll (barbecueroll).

Appiani/Goufani Maneavoure

It is performed for Lat canalithiasis. Lie the patient on their side so that the affected side is facing upwards. Wait for one minute or till Nystagmus subsides. Then quickly turn patient's head downwards to look at the floor. Keep in this position for one minute or till the nystagmus subsides.

Cupulolithiasis (Horizontal Canal)

- Prolonged attacks. Can be for more than 2–3 minutes.
- Horizontal nystagmus on either side. May be stronger on the affected side.
- Otoconia get stuck to the cupula of the canal.

- Treatment is the same as the lateral canal. Try a head shake for 30seconds before starting the manoeuvre.
- Semont's manoeuvre can be very useful.

Semont's Manevoeure

- Ask the patient to sit on the edge of the bed and turn the head to one side. Put a pillow on one end of the bed.
- Now hold the patient's head gently and lie him down with head facing upwards (looking at the ceiling) on the opposite end of the bed where the pillow is.
- Put your hand on the patient's forehead and swiftly swing patient to other end of bed so the face comes in contact with the pillow.
- The important thing to remember is to perform this rather quickly and firmly so that the patient's face almost bangs on the pillow. This sudden bang can dislodge the crystals (e.g., in cupulolithiasis).

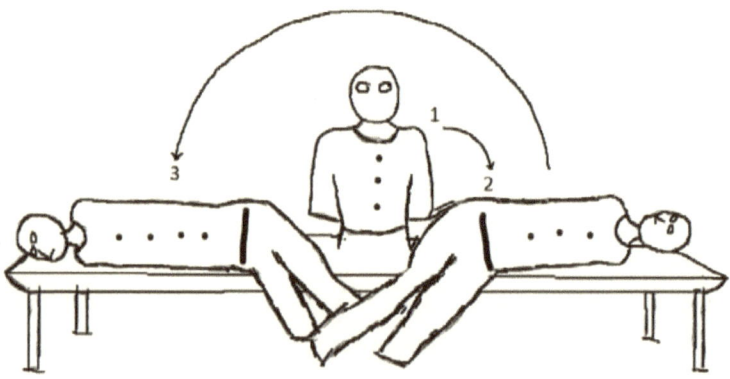

Figure 13. Semont's Manoeuvre.

Vertebral Artery Occlusion/Vertebro Basilar Insufficiency/Cervical Vertigo

- It is a rare cause. Formina are widened due to pulsation of artery, so symptoms only occur in extreme head positions.

- May be history to trauma(whiplash).
- Difficult to diagnose. It is a diagnosis of exclusion.
- Angiography is needed if vascular cause is to be excluded.
- Treatment is usually treatment of the cause.

Clinically, there may be different scenarios that may be encountered.

Negative Hallpike or Subjectively Positive Hallpike with Classical History

- This may be due to the fact that nystagmus is fatigable.
- Sometimes it is so subtle that it may not be recognised by the naked eye. (Frenzel glass or VNG can be useful.)
- It is recommended to do the test early in the morning if possible.
- Even in cases where nystagmus is not visible but Hallpike is subjectively positive, Epley should be done on the affected side.

Anxiety

- Patients sometimes do not allow carrying out the Hallpike or Epley due to their fear of sickness.
- Reassure the patient and reappoint at some other time.
- Surgery

This is not the favoured mode of treatment. It is done only in exceptionally rare cases which have failed the conventional treatment.

- Partial or complete plugging of post canal.
- Transection of posterior ampullary nerve.

Carefully selected cases in good hands show good results from these types of surgeries.

Management Balance Disorders in Elderly Patients

ᘓᘔ

Dizziness is the tenthmost common issue in primary care. Almost 10 per cent of patients present with this problem. Studies have shown that 30 per cent of the population by the age of sixty-five years can suffer with the balance disorders, and out of them,one in ten ends up with handicapping dizziness.

In the primary care setup, dizziness can be a dilemma, especially in the elderly population. The majority of these patients have pre-existing comorbidities and age-related issues. Commonly, first assessment does not provide enough clues towards any diagnosis. The initial presentation can be quite dramatic, and more sinister issues like CVA need to be ruled out. Constraints of time and resources make it a challenging task. Assessment of complex, multifactorial, and long-term chronic issues may need thorough clinical evaluation and possible balance lab tests to reach a diagnosis. This will not be in the remit of primary care physicians.

As we know, there are three basic components of balance control.

1. Sensory input (visual, peripheral vestibular system, and from joint and muscular tissues)
2. Integration of sensation within the central nervous system
3. Performing motor commands

Physiologically, each of the components shows some loss of function with age. This may be due to generalised vascular changes, ischaemia, and atrophic changes. In addition, certain disease processes (e.g.,diabetes) or iatrogenic factors can also play an important role. There is also deterioration in functional abilities (e.g., decrease in muscle strength, sensory perception) and decrease in motor responsiveness. This will result in diminished compensatory response and hence poor balance control in these patients.

Direct insults to the balance system (e.g.,labyrinthitis) are not uncommon in elderly patients. The natural compensation is compromised in the majority of patients, so spontaneous recovery from vestibular failure can be quite difficult. Due to the decline in physiologic abilities and existing comorbidities in many cases, even vestibular rehabilitation may be of limited benefit. This can be attributed to many different reasons such as associated ailments, the general physical condition, and the social support (e.g., an elderly patient living alone with little or no family support will be very difficult to rehabilitate). Needless to say,a well-resourced physiotherapy department will be able to provide better care to the patients in general.

Common Causes of Dizziness in Elderly

		Presentation	Causes
1	Physiologic Ageing	Mild imbalance	Age-related decline in sensory, vestibular, or motor functions
2	Musculoskeletal Disorders	Imbalance	Arthritis, myopathies, proprioceptive issues
3	BPPV	Typically short-lived attacks when turns in bed or looks up or down.	Calcium carbonate crystals (otoconia) move from the utricle to the semicircular canals

4	Orthostatic Hypotension	Brief episodes of dizziness. May complain of fainting upon standing up and relieved by sitting or lying.	Drop of systolic BP (≥20mmHg). Commonly drug related
5	Neurological	True vertigo or imbalance with associated other neurological symptoms (e.g.,neuropathies, cranial nerve involvements)	CVA, Parkinson's,peripheral neuropathies (DM)
6	Cardiac	Brief episodes of dizziness/ fainting associated with palpitations or bradycardia	Cardiac arrythmia
7	Drug Related	Feeling of constant imbalance or true vertigo, which could be episodic.	There can be a variety of reasons (e.g.,ototoxicity, vestibular sedation, hypoglycemia)

Dizziness should be regarded as a significant symptom in the elderly. It can have a major impact on their daily routine (in terms of their ability to look after themselves) and on their carers.

It can lead to social isolation because they will be frightened to mobilise independently due to risks of falling. They may develop anxiety and depression. In many situations, this can lead to further deterioration in the balance disorders. In order to avoid the situation going into a downwards spiral, early intervention in these cases is of paramount importance.

Surprisingly, a large number of elderly patients can be either treated successfully or adequately rehabilitated to lead relatively symptom-free lives.

Assessment of Elderly Patients with Dizziness

History is by far the most important aspect of assessment. A large number of the elderly patients present with more than one sensation of dizziness. The presentation may be a combination of spinning, light-headedness, and off balance, and they may have a history of falls. History of the associated symptoms is essential because these symptoms can be subtle and may not have been previously reported by the patient. The review of the systems should be broad and must include enquiries about vision, hearing, arthritis, neck pain, neuropathies, and cardiovascular issues. Polypharmacy (e.g.,antiepileptics, barbiturates, antipsychotic medicines, and diuretics) are important drugs to be considered carefully. It is very important to enquire about functional status of patients and the severity of impact they are experiencing on their daily activities.

Clinical examination in the elderly will depend on the presentation. In a typical history of BPPV, one may not need to go ahead with exhaustive clinical and audiological tests. On the other hand, it is imperative to perform the Hallpike test in all elderly patients irrespective of their presentation.

It is also essential that a complete and accurate clinical examination of gait and stance is performed. It is useful to evaluate spontaneous gait of elderly patients along with the size of the base of support. Other clinical elementary tests can be performed. In the 'timed up-and-go' test, the patient is simply asked to stand up, walk three meters, turn, walk back, and sit down again. People taking longer than thirty seconds are classified as physically dependent, whereas those taking less than twenty seconds are considered normal.

Cognitive and psychiatric assessment should be done to identify the cognitive deficit of dementia and to evaluate whether there are any symptoms of depression.

Two of the most important factors in elderly patient's assessment are:

1. To establish the degree of disability they are experiencing due to balance problems.

This is not an easy task. Many varying factors are intertwined in it. These include pre-existing medical conditions and social and psychological issues.

2. Falls.

   This may be single most fearful factor for an elderly patient. They lose confidence and can become socially reclusive. They become afraid to carry out even the simplest tasks. This can lead to a further deterioration in balance disorders and may result in a downward vicious cycle. Specific predisposing factors like sequel of stroke (hemiparesis), Parkinson's, myolpathies, or polyneuropathies need to be recognised early. Involvement of other disciples like a falls team is very important.

Investigations of these patients should be outlined in light of the presentation and associated comorbidities. There will not be any need to subject most of these patients to the exhaustive battery of balance lab tests. It will be more appropriate to concentrate on the related issues (e.g., cardiovascular, musculoskeletal, neurological, or polypharmacy).

Treatment of Elderly Patients with Dizziness

Their pre-existing ailments (e.g., musculoskeletal or neurological) may be aggravated by the vestibular issue. These patients also develop unrealistic expectations of the outcome of treatment. Counselling the patients and detailed discussion of the management of their condition will form the basis of the treatment. Involvement of other disciples should always be considered,such asa falls team. They are usually community-based teams of physiotherapists, social workers, and occupational health care individuals. They assess the patients in their own environment and work towards making it safe for them to mobilise. Simple modifications like hand rails in corridors or stairs, hand grips in bathtubs or showers, and identifying hazards in the house (e.g., rugs, ill-fitting carpets) will significantly reduce the risk of falls.

Involvement of cardiology or neurology teams can greatly improve the care of patients.

In elderly patients, vestibular rehabilitation can play a major role. The vestibular therapist will need to look at a very broad picture. Due to age- or disease-related deterioration of physiological abilities, one needs to look globally to help patients. For example, to stabilise the gait in these patients, the therapist will have to improve proprioception and look into using substitution methods. Patients may need persuasion and training to use walking aids.

It is of paramount importance to look into the patient's psychological issues. Elderly patients often suffer with depression or anxiety issues for a variety of reasons. Recognising and addressing these issues will help hugely in the long-term management of these patients.

An important aspect of treatment will be the provision of social care for these patients at their home and in the communities. It will be almost impossible to achieve favourable results in the absence of this kind of infrastructure. Simple steps like home help (either by family or social services) and integrating them in a social network can result in an immensely positive outcome for these patients.

Dizziness in Children

෴

Dizziness is an uncommon condition in children, and it can be a challenging task to manage. Vertigo can be associated with a number of different syndromes in children. It is useful to divide the balance problems in children with hearing loss and vertigo and dizziness. The common causes of dizziness in children are as follows.

1. Otitis media (acute/chronic suppurative)
2. Otologic conditions like congenital perilymph fistula
3. Otitis media with effusion (glue ears)
4. Migraine-associated vertigo
5. BPVC (benign paroxysmal vertigo of childhood)
6. BPPV (benign paroxysmal positional vertigo)
7. Brain injuries or tumours
8. Psychological (usually in teens)

About 2–5 per cent of children suffer with vertigo symptoms. Only 33 per cent of them will have a diagnosis. Patients with developmental delays, those with a family history of migraine, and teenagers are more likely to develop balance problems.

The commonest cause of dizziness in children is BPVC. This is considered as a migraine equivalent. It can occur in 35 per cent of all children presenting with balance issues. There are short episodes of vertigo with no aural symptoms, and it is not positional. There are no precipitating factors. It is prevalent from four to twelve years of age. A large majority of children with this condition go on to develop migraines in later life. This condition is not the same as BPPV of adults. BPPV is positional and is due to presence of otoconia in semicircular canals, whereas BPVC is a migraine variant.

Assessment of a Dizzy Child

Dizziness is a vague term that includes light-headedness, anxiety, ataxia, visual disturbance, hyperventilation, weakness, depression, and true vertigo. It is difficult for young children to describe their symptoms, making the evaluation challenging. However, a thorough history and physical examination can establish a diagnosis in most cases.

History of dizziness in children should include perinatal history of infection, drugs,and family history of migraine, epilepsy, and neurological conditions like MS. Recognition of syndromes and craniofacial abnormalities are important.

Presenting symptoms in a child also differ. They can present with clumsiness, falls, or episodes which children or the parents may describe as frightening, where they have to clutch the nearest object. There may be abnormal behaviour or delayed response as well.

Examination of children will need patience and practice. It may not be possible in a routine, busy clinic. Assessment of gait, posture,and the oculomotor system will be done as in adults, but one will have to innovate ways to do these tests in a child.

Look at the children to see how they manage to walk and maintain gait. Involve them in play with toys to see the level of coordination. It is important to make a note of their developmental landmarks. Specialist paediatric balance clinics where facilities and trained staff is available will be the most useful.

It is difficult to plan a universal scheme of investigations for a young child with balance problems. There will be huge variations due to age factor, behavioural issues, and developmental status of child, as well as parents' or carers' concerns and level of understanding the problem.

Routine haematology including FBC and TSH is important. Balance lab tests (VNG) can be done for the child depending on the age and cooperation of the child.

Treatment

Treatment of balance problems in children is a challenging task, to say the least. The commonest problem affecting the age group of four to five years is BPVC. This is a migraine variant and is self-limiting in the majority of individuals. In severe cases, the management will be the same as a vestibular migraine. It will include prevention and medical therapy of the migraine, and there may be vestibular rehabilitation.

Vestibular rehabilitation in children needs a lot more customization than in adults. It needs innovative ways and techniques to integrate in simple and fun methods (e.g., modifying their toys or play methods). One useful way is to use balance boards or video games that use hand/eye coordination. These should be under supervision and have a thought-over process on addressing the underlying balance issue.

It is important to consider the environmental factors thoroughly because there will be huge implications of these factors in children. It is not only the child but the parents who have to be aware of risks and of health and safety factors in implementing daily tasks. It could be quite a daunting task for the parents to be conscious of the child's safety at all times. They will have to be trained in how to supervise safety in activities like swimming or even playing in the park with other children.

Vestibular Rehabilitation

The concept of vestibular rehabilitation for patients with balance disorders is very old. In 1944, physician Dr Cawthorne and therapist Mr Cooksey noticed that patients with brain injuries who mobilised early got better quicker. They developed a programme of exercises to formally help these patients, and it was a great success. These exercise regimes, termed Cawthorne Cooksey exercises, are still employed in balance physiotherapy.

It was not until 1993 when Szturm and Kreb discovered that there was dramatic improvement in patient symptoms when they customised the exercises according to the individual patient.

Later on, eminent physiotherapist Susan Herdman did a lot of work on patients with balance disorders and has made a huge contribution in this field. Her work was instrumental in incorporating the different methods of vestibular rehabilitation into day-to-day activities. She helped to develop customised regimes by using many unconventional methods (e.g., using a treadmill in front of a large screen TV displaying varying images and videos).

There are many studies which have proven that customised and supervised exercises have a superior outcome in balance rehabilitation.

Nature has a very efficient way of utilizing compensatory mechanisms in the event of vestibular failure to keep the body's balance system in check. The vestibular organs do not regenerate when damaged, but the patient does not remain unstable throughout life.

Balance is maintained in the body by the vestibular system, which through semicircular canals (by sensing angular motion) and otolithic organs (linear, gravity-related motions) produces postural control and oculomotor responses. These responses are modified by the higher centres, like the cerebellum and cortical areas of the brain, to fully integrate the body's response to a given task according to particular situation, time, and place.

All these systems work seamlessly at the subconscious level. In situations where deficiency is encountered at any level, either peripheral (vestibular organs, propriocetive, visual) or central (cerebellum or cortical) compensatory processes automatically come into play. Patients with vestibular failure start to use more visual cues (they find it very difficult to walk in dark areas), or they rely more on sensory inputs from joints or feet. It becomes difficult for them to maintain the balance and posture control on uneven floors or stairs.

There is huge plasticity in all these systems,and they can be successfully manipulated by appropriate rehabilitation techniques in treatment balance disorders.

Vestibular rehabilitation therapy acts in three ways.
1. Adaptation: Improper signals from damaged vestibular organ create unwanted retinal slip (image slipping from fovea to periphery), leading to destabilization of gaze. The brain learns to adapt changes in vestibular signals. In most patients, this adaptation will occur spontaneously. However, in some cases it has to be achieved by specific exercises.
2. Habituation: Mismatched sensory input is an important cause of balance problems. Error situations are repetitively

presented to the brain so that it habituates (conditions) itself and reduces symptoms.

3. Compensation/Substitution: The partial or total loss of function in one organ is taken over by other senses (e.g., visual or proprioceptive). The improper signals are overruled by other senses. The compensation can be spontaneous, but it will most effectively be achieved by vestibular rehabilitation therapy.

Goals of Vestibular Rehabilitation

1. The main aim is to improve the patient's functional ability to keep balance in control in both static and ambulatory situations.
2. Improve the patient's general condition of balance by working on techniques of postural stability. This will reduce the risk of fall and increase the patient's confidence. It will also work towards improving the patient's general physical condition.
3. Improve the patient's psychological profile so that effective social integration can take place.

Assessment of Patients for Vestibular Rehabilitation

There is a conventional understanding that vestibular rehabilitation does not work for fluctuant vestibular issues. This is largely true but not a hard and fast rule. For example, patients with Ménière's and uncompensated vestibular deficit, or patients with vestibular migraine with strong vestibular overlay, will benefit from rehabilitation measures as much as patients with fixed vestibular disorders. Patients with these disorders will need medical therapy in conjunction with rehab.

In complex cases where it is difficult to reach a definite diagnosis of vestibular failure, vestibular rehabilitation can be started, and it has been reported to have positive effects.

A thorough assessment of balance issues and diagnosis of the underlying condition is mandatory before the start of the rehabilitation programme. It is of paramount importance to bear in mind the associated problems which may be pre-existing (e.g., spinal problems, arthritis) or problems resulting from vestibular involvement (e.g.,musculoskeletal, posture, and psychological issues). Rehabilitation programmes which do not integrate all the above factors may not be successful.

There are three main areas of assessment.
1. Functional Assessment: This will be based on standard balance tests in a clinic situation (e.g.,gait, posture, coordination).
2. Symptoms: Trigger factors (e.g.,visual, mobility, and certainsituations like crowded areas andsupermarkets).
3. System: Pre-existing conditions like arthritis (especially in cervical spine), CNS lesions, and visual or musculoskeletal disorders. Drugs andpsychiatric issues which may be pre-existing or may have developed secondary to balance problems must not be overlooked. Age is also an important factor.

These will not only help to effectively customise the therapy but will also establish a realistic outcome for a particular individual. It will clarify the goals and expectations of patients and the therapist.

It is good practice to ask patients to score their feelings and symptoms on a chart called the Dizziness Handicap Inventory (DHI). It is a subjective scoring system but can become a useful tool during the course of therapy to assess the progress of the patient as the score decreases with an improvement in symptoms. It can also be used to objectively reassure patients about their progress.

Dizziness Handicap Inventory

P	1.	Does looking up increase your symptoms?	o	Yes
			o	No
			o	Sometimes
E	2.	Do you feel frustrated because of your problem?	o	Yes
			o	No
			o	Sometimes
F	3.	Do you restrict your travel for business and recreation? -	o	Yes
			o	No
			o	Sometimes
P	4.	Does walking down the aisle of a supermarket increase your problem?	o	Yes
			o	No
			o	Sometimes
F	5.	Do you have difficulty getting into or out of bed?	o	Yes
			o	No
			o	Sometimes
F	6.	Does your problem significantly restrict your participation in social activities (e.g.,going out for dinners, movies, dancing)?	o	Yes
			o	No
			o	Sometimes
F	7.	Do have difficulty in reading because of your problem?	o	Yes
			o	No
			o	Sometimes
P	8.	Does performing more ambitious activities such as sports, dancing, and household work increase your problem?	o	Yes
			o	No
			o	Sometimes
E	9.	Are you afraid to leave your home unaccompanied because of your problem?	o	Yes
			o	No
			o	Sometimes
E	10.	Have you felt embarrassed because of your problem?	o	Yes
			o	No
			o	Sometimes

P	11. Do quick movements of your head increase your problem?	o	Yes
		o	No
		o	Sometimes
F	12. Do you avoid heights because of your problem?	o	Yes
		o	No
		o	Sometimes
P	13. Does turning over in bed increases your problem?	o	Yes
		o	No
		o	Sometimes
E	14. Are you afraid people may think you are intoxicated?	o	Yes
		o	No
		o	Sometimes
F	15. It is difficult for you to do home or yard work because of your problem?	o	Yes
		o	No
		o	Sometimes
F	16. Is it difficult for you to go to walk by yourself because of your problem?	o	Yes
		o	No
		o	Sometimes
F	17. Is walking down a sidewalk a problem for you?	o	Yes
		o	No
		o	Sometimes
E	18. Is it difficult for you to concentrate because of your problem?	o	Yes
		o	No
		o	Sometimes
F	19. Is it difficult for you to walk around the house in the dark?	o	Yes
		o	No
		o	Sometimes
E	20. Are you afraid to stay home alone because of your problem?	o	Yes
		o	No
		o	Sometimes
E	21. Do you feel handicapped because of your problem?	o	Yes
		o	No
		o	Sometimes
E	22. Has this problem placed stress in relationship with family and friends?	o	Yes
		o	No
		o	Sometimes
E	23. Are you depressed because of this problem?	o	Yes
		o	No
		o	Sometimes

F	24. Does this problem interfere with your job and household responsibilities?	o	Yes
		o	No
		o	Sometimes
P	25. Does bending over increase your problem?	o	Yes
		o	No
		o	Sometimes

Scoring :

Yes=4, No= 0, Sometimes=2

Maximum score is 100. Minimum score is 0.

16–34= Mild handicap

35–52 = Moderate handicap

Above 53 = Severe handicap

All patients above 10 should be referred to balance specialists.

P= Physical, F= Functional, E= Emotional

Evaluation	Physical	Emotional	Functional	Total Score
Reassess 1				
Reassess 2				
Reassess 3				
Reassess 4				

The patient is assessed on the above guidelines, physician's diagnosis, and the balance tests (VNG/calorics, and computerised dynamic posturography if available). The plans for VRT (vestibular rehabilitation) are then customised in order to effectively treat the issue.

The principals of VRT revolve around training and building up methods of adaptation, habituation, and compensation/substitution in daily life. The baseline aims of vestibular rehabilitation are:

1. Stabilise the gaze.
2. Stabilise posture and gait.
3. Desensitization of trigger factors.

These broad principals are employed for patients after assessment and weighting them in accordance with their individual presentation and circumstances. This approach can be understood as customization. As we know from the wide variation in a patient's presentation and circumstances, the response of VRT is quite varied. Nature has provided an innate ability for the human body to compensate so that a large majority of patients get almost back to normal spontaneously. However, there are almost 20–30 per cent of patients who continue to have problems of varying severity which may affect their daily lives. Vestibular issues affect almost 45 per cent of the general population above forty-five years of age, and so it constitutes a large number of people.

1. Gaze Stabilization

Gaze stabilization is by far the most important of all the rehabilitation therapies. Vestibulo ocular reflex (VOR) stabilises the gaze during head movements. All objects around us are always kept in sharp focus irrespective of whether head the is static or moving. It works by moving the eyes at the same speed as the head movement but in the opposite direction.

The clearest image of any object is formed in the centre of the fovea. During any motion, the image slips to the periphery, causing it to blur. Movement of two degrees from centre will lead to a 50 per cent decrease in visual acuity.

To keep the image in the centre of the fovea, the eyes make corrective motions called nystagmus, which has a slow and a quick phase. VOR keeps the image central with the slow phase of eye (opposite to head movements).

In patients with vestibular disorders, VOR is affected in most cases. This leads to destabilization of the gaze-fixing mechanism, and patients find their mobility is compromised, especially in high-velocity head movements (e.g.,walking, running, and turning). It can even affect the visual acuity. In patients with vestibular failure, the visual acuity can drop up to four lines.

VOR exercises are established to stabilise the gaze and increase gain of the vestibular system. It is done by retraining the VOR (vestibulo ocular reflex)and VSR (vestibulo spinal reflex) mechanisms to improve the adaptation. Commonly, it is the first set of exercises given to patients. It is important to explain to patients that these measures will bring back some symptoms, and that is quite normal. Unless there are significant symptoms, they should continue. Perseverance is the key. Example exercises are as follows.

a. Fix eyes to a stationary object (about a metre away) and move head right and left. Do it for ten seconds and increase upto thirty seconds. Initially do it while sitting, and make sure the background behind is plain and not busy (e.g.,patterned curtains). After this, repeat while standing, followed by doing it while walking a few steps. Patients can do it two to three times per day and build it up as symptoms get better.

b. Move eyes right, left,up, and down on a target with the head in a fixed neutral position. Repeat in the same way as above.

These exercises are performed using small targets (for foveal stimulation) and large targets (for full field stimulation). The head movements can be in either the horizontal or vertical direction. It is important to explain to patients what to expect in generalised terms.

2. Gait and Posture Stabilization

Functional balance is a fine interaction between maintaining centre of gravity (COG) above the base of support in static or dynamic situations. Base of support is the area of contact between feet and the surface. Strategies to acquire balance control will be determined by the stability of the patient or the nature of the base of support (e.g., firm, mobile, rough, or smooth)because these will alter the area of contact with the feet. Sensory deficits will have the same effect as well.

We resist falling by constantly altering our COG relative to the base of support. In cases where there are excessive movements of surface, we step forward or backwards. Sudden changes in movements of the surface may cause stumbling.

During our day-to-day lives, we experience constantly changing base of support. The body applies three basic strategies to maintain COG in relation to base of support.
*   Ankle Strategy

When the base is firm and COG movements are slow, rotation of the body takes place about ankle joint as a rigid mass.
*   Hip Strategy

When movements of the trunk are rapid or the base of support is unpredictable, large movements at the hip are necessary.
*   Step Strategy

With a very large shift in body position or excessive movement of the base of support, a step is required to widen the base of support.

Age factors and pre-existing musculoskeletal, neurological, and other medical ailments are important to consider in the initial evaluation.

Evaluation should start with assessment of gait, posture, and the methods which the patient uses to mobilise (e.g., what support is needed to stand up, whether walking sticks or a frame is used).

A patient who develops gait and/or posture instability will need to develop substitution or compensatory strategies to replace the lost vestibular functions. Gaze stabilization alone may not be sufficient.

These patients will need instruction to work on developing appropriate posture (e.g., in the elderly or people with CNS disorder) or tasks to improve the control of their centre of gravity by coordinating ankle, hip, or step strategies. For example, use of parallel bars, standing close to a wall (for patients who have fear of falling), reaching or lifting, throwing, standing on narrow beam, or tandem walk. All of these can be customised by the physiotherapist, or patients can be trained to customise themselves according to their symptoms and environment. It is important to explain to patients that the best outcome will be achieved if these strategies are approached in a steady, progressive manner. That means when they become symptom-free during a task, they will need to slightly alter it to make it more challenging. For example, if they have no issue standing tandem, try with closed eyes, change the base of support, or stand on a softer or narrower support.

This is where instruction and training from a trained balance physiotherapist will benefit the patients.

Patients must be made aware that rehabilitation is a slow and tedious process. It needs a lot of perseverance, constant input from health professionals, and at times moral and psychological support within the community and family support.

3. Desensitization of Trigger Factors

Many patients with vestibular disorders develop oversensitivity to certain stimulus. They are usually visually evoked. It happens when a sensory mismatch develops between vestibular, spinal, and musculoskeletal systems. These patients will become excessively dizzy in situations where complex visual inputs are likely, such assupermarkets, driving, and patterned surroundings (floors, walls, fabric). It is imperative to recognise this entity because it can be treated quite effectively and may result in dramatic improvement in a patient's symptoms. Failure to appreciate it will result in an unsatisfactory outcome of VRT.

The patient's visual sensitivity can be decreased by repeated optokinetic stimuli. This can be achieved by clever manipulation of day-to-day activities. There may be no need for any expensive set up to help patients. For example,starting to walk inrelatively quiet areas and then going in larger town centres or busy supermarkets can be a simple, practical, and effective way for these patients to start a retraining programme. These simple tasks can be made interesting by small but meaningful innovations to increase their effectiveness. Asking the patient to hold a trolley first with both hands and look right and left in busy aisles, and then let go of the trolley. Carefully selected video games, virtual reality sets, and interactive video games where hand/eye coordination, or even balance boards, are used.

These are all different ways to innovate and customise patients' VRT. Primarily, it will be based on the objectives we have discussed above (i.e.,stabilization of gaze, posture, and desensitization of triggers).

As we can see, changing and altering pathways according to need and the patient's environment will increase the patient's interest and involvement. This can result ina hugely positive outcome during rehabilitation.

References

1. Al Mohiza Mohd., Quality improvement in Balance and rehabilitation and its effect on Quality of life J Neurol Phys Ther,40/2 (April 2016), 156.
2. Susan Herdman, 'Advances in the Treatment of Vestibular Disorders', *J. Physical Therapy*,77/6 (June 1997), 602–618.
3. Thomas Brandt, Andreas Zwergal, Michael Strupp, 'Medical Treatment of Vestibular Disorders'1537–1548,published online (15 June 2009).
4. Susan J. Herdman, 'Treatment of Vestibular Disorders in Traumatically Brain-injured Patients', *Journal of Head Trauma Rehabilitation* (December 1990).
5. Akinori Itoh and Eiji Sakata,'Treatment of Vestibular Disorders',617–623,published online (8 July 2009).
6. Adolf Bronstein and Thomas Lamport, "Dizziness: A Practical Approach to Diagnosis and Management". Published 2007, Cambridge University Press
7. Joel Goebel, Practical Management of the Dizzy Patient. Published 1991, Lippencot
8. Efficacy and Safety of Betahistine Treatment in Patients with Ménière'sDisease: Primary Results of a Long Term, Multicentre, Double Blind, Randomised, Placebo Controlled, Dose Defining Trial (BEMED trial)', *BMJ* (21 January 2016), 352.
9. F Lezius, C Adrion, U Mansmann, K Jahn, M Strupp, 'High-dosage Betahistine Dihydrochloride between 288 and 480

mg/Day in Patients with Severe Menière's Disease: ACase Series'. Eur Arch Otorhinolaryngol (2011) 268:1237–1240

10. Current Opinion in Neurobiology 1994, Review Journal.

11. Serafina Chimirri,Rossana Aiello, 'Verigo/Dizziness as Adverse Drug Reactions',*Journal of Pharmacology & Therapeutics*(December 2013).

12. Cochrane Database of Systematic Reviews:. Modifications of the Epley Manoeuvre for Benign Paroxysmal Positional Vertigo (BPPV).

13. American Hearing Research Foundation., Management Of Balance Disorders

14. Vestibular Disorder Association,educational resources.

15. S A MacKeith, O J Whiteside, T Mawby, I D Bottrill, 'Middle Ear Gentamicin-soaked Pledgets in the Treatment of Ménière's Disease', *Otoneuro* (February 2014).

16. 'Vertigo/Dizziness as Drug's Adverse Reaction', *J Pharmaciol Pharmacother*(December 2013).

17. Jeremy Skoog, *Vestibular Rehabilitation*, YouTube.

18. Matthe Coleman, 'Breaking News: Treating Vestibular Disorders Is Child's Play',*The Hearing Journal*, 64/12 (December 2011),10.

19. Mitesh Patel, Kiran Agarwal, Qadeer Arshad, Mohamed Hariri, Peter Rea,M Seemungal, John F Golding, Jonny P Harcourt, 'Intratympanic Methylprednisolone versus Gentamicin in Patients with Unilateral Ménière's',(16 November 2016)

20. Ann Med Health Sci Res. 2014 Jan-Feb; 4(1): 3–7. doi: 10.4103/2141-9248.126601The Influence of Psychological Factors in Meniere's Disease

Index

cochlear hydrops 51
Cogan's syndrome 50
cognitive 85
computerised dynamic posturography (CPD) 35
counselling 47,54,63,78,86
cupulolithiasis 74,76,79,80

D
dark cell theory 51
desensitization 98,102
Dix Hallpike 21,28,75,76
drop attacks 51

E
electronystagmography 25
electrocochleography 53
endolypmphatic system 51
endolymphatic sac 51
endolymphatic duct 51
endolymphatic succus decompression 64
Epley 75,76,77

F
food triggers for migrane 67
Frenzel glasses 15,17,43

G
gait 18,100
gaze-evoked nystagmus 17
gaze control system 4
gaze stabilization 98
Gentamicin 60,61,62
geotropic nystagmus 76
goufani 79

H
head shake 18,21,80
head thrust 18
hemiplegic gait 19
hip strategy 8,36,100
horizontal canal (lateral canal) 2,4,25,28,29,30,31,37,

I
idiopathic endolymphatic hydrops 50

L
labrynthitis 45,50
Leromoyez syndrome 51
log roll 79

M
mal de barquement syndrome 48
Meniere's 50
Meniett device 63
methyleprednisolone 58
migraine associated vertigo 52
myopathic gait 19

N
neuropathic gait 19

O
ocular motor 27
ocular sign 45
ocular system 6
orthostatic hypotension 14,84
otolithic crises 51,61
otolithic organ 3,4,99
ototoxicity 84

V

www.ingramcontent.com/pod-product-compliance
Lightning Source LLC
Chambersburg PA
CBHW050356290526

45786CB00003B/1015